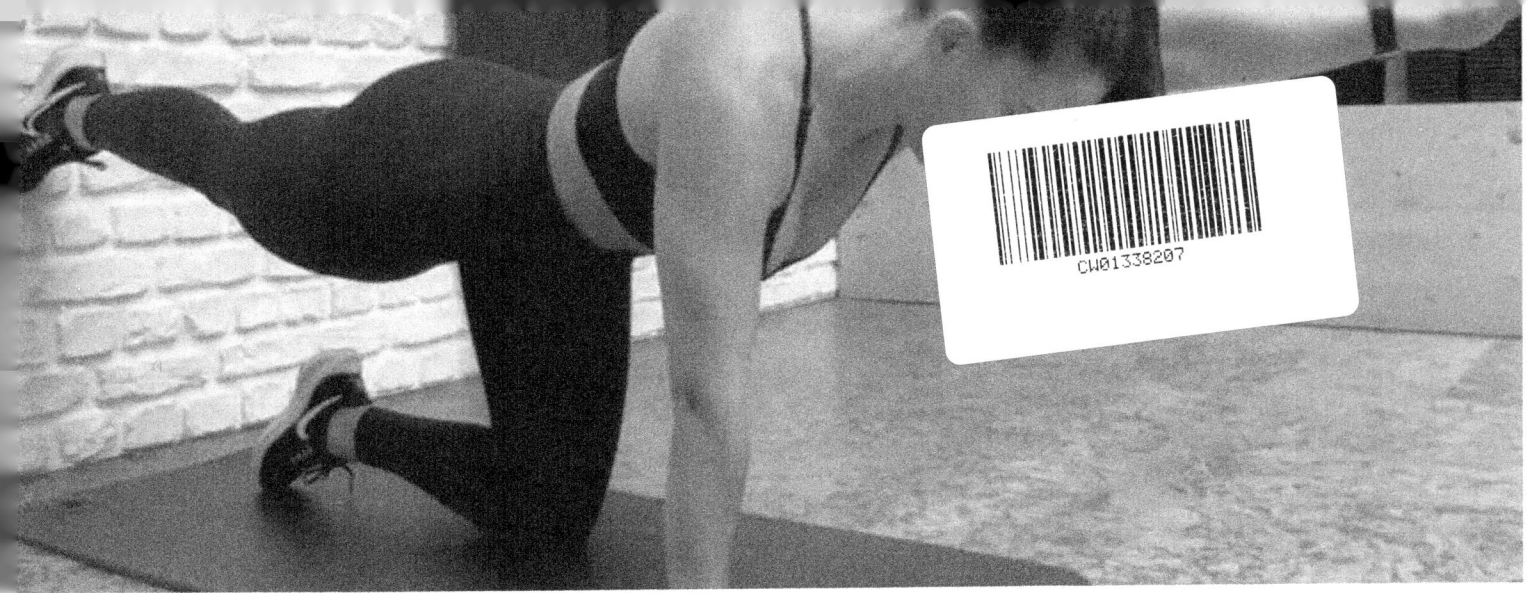

WALL PILATES
For Women

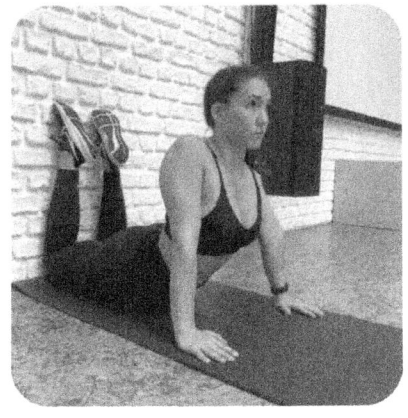
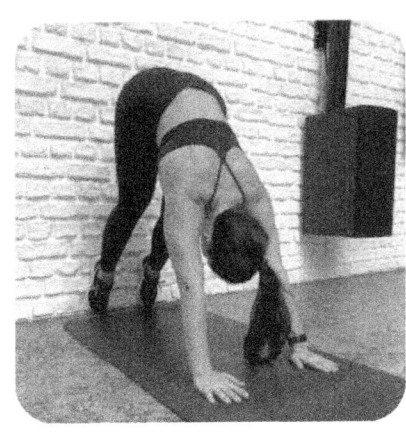
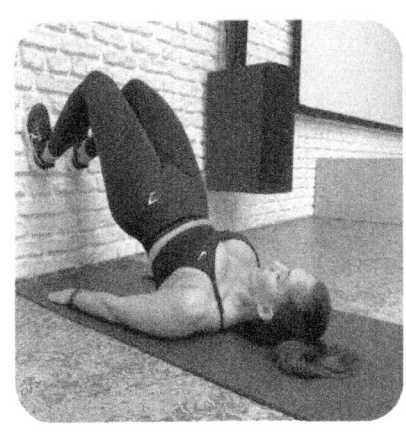

FLEXIBILITY **BALANCE** **STRENGTH**

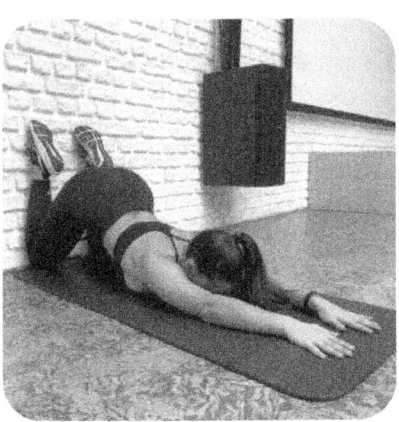
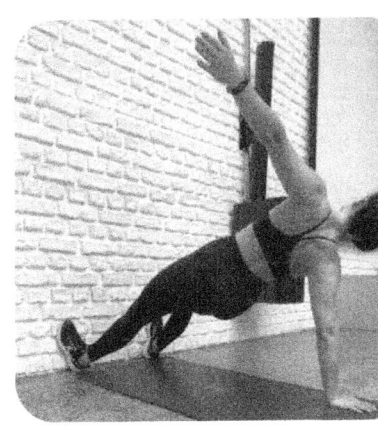
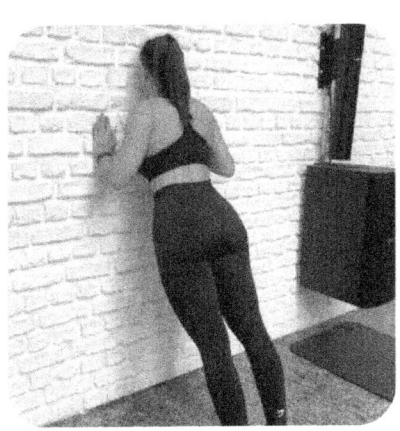

Eva Ross

© Copyright 2023 - All rights reserved by **Eva Ross**

The content contained within this book may not be reproduced, duplicated or transmitted without direct written permission from the author or the publisher.

Under no circumstances will any blame or legal responsibility be held against the publisher, or author, for any damages, reparation, or monetary loss due to the information contained within this book, either directly or indirectly.

Legal Notice:

This book is copyright protected. It is only for personal use. You cannot amend, distribute, sell, use, quote or paraphrase any part, or the content within this book, without the consent of the author or publisher.

Disclaimer Notice:

Please note the information contained within this document is for educational and entertainment purposes only. All effort has been executed to present accurate, up to date, reliable, complete information. No warranties of any kind are declared or implied. Readers acknowledge that the author is not engaged in the rendering of legal, financial, medical or professional advice. The content within this book has been derived from various sources. Please consult a licensed professional before attempting any techniques outlined in this book.

TABLE OF CONTENTS

INTRODUCTION 5

CHAPTER 1: WALL PILATES: WHAT YOU REALLY NEED 7
   EQUIPMENT AND TOOLS 7
   SPACE REQUIREMENTS & PRACTICE AREA 8
   SET YOUR GOALS 10

CHAPTER 2: SAFETY AND PRECAUTIONS 13

CHAPTER 3: WARM-UP AND COOLDOWN 17
   THE IMPORTANCE OF WARM-UP 17
   WARM-UP EXERCISES 19
      Wall Mountain Climbers 20
      Wall Lateral Lunges 21
      Wall Leg Swings 22
      Wall Single-Leg Lifts 23
      Wall Calf Raises 24
      Arm Circles 25
      Wall Single Leg Circles 26
      Wall Angels 27
      Knee To Nose 28
      Wall Leg Raise + Kick Back 29
   COOLDOWN EXERCISES 31
      Wall Cobra Pose 33
      Wall Cat Pose 34
      Lower Body Stretch 35
      Wall-Assisted Puppy Pose 36
      Wall Sphinx Pose 37

CHAPTER 4: COMPREHENSIVE WALL PILATES EXERCISES 39
   ABS & CORE EXERCISES 39
      Abs And Core Crunch Version 40
      Abs And Core Oblique Version 41
      Wall Bicycle Crunches 42
      Wall Pike Crunches 43
      Wall Abdominal Press Legs Version 44
      Superman 45
      Wall Teaser Abs Core 46
      Wall Walking Plank 47
      Dolphine Pose 48
      Dolphine Pose With Feet Elevated On Wall 49
      Reverse Curl 50

ARMS & SHOULDERS STRETCHES AND STRENGHTING EXERCISES 51
Arm Bends 52
Arms/Shoulder Stretch 53
Wall Push-Ups 54
Wall Push-Ups Dog Pose Version 55
Seated Trunk Rotation 56
Wall Touches Plank 57
Extended Downward Plank 58

LOWER BODY EXERCISES 59
Wall Hip Thrust / Bridge With Both Legs 60
Lunges Classic 61
Lunges + Kick Back 62
Back To The Wall Lunges 63
Wall Squats 64
Wall Sit Heel Raise 65
Standing Wall Leg Lift 66
Clamshells 67
Forward Wall Squats 68
One-Legged Wall Sit 69
Glute Bridge Half-Assisted 70
Single Leg Glute Bridge 71

FLEXIBILITY AND BALANCE EXERCISES 73
Wall Side Leg Lift 74
Toe Touch Crunch 75
Wall Table Tob 76
Wall Single Leg Stretch (Left & Right) 77
Wall Scissor 78
Extended Glute Bridge Rotation 79
Dynamic Plank With Wall Support 80

CHAPTER 5: SPECIALIZED WORKOUT PROGRAMS 81
Warm Up Routine (10 Mins) 81
Cooldown Routine 83
Flexibility Focus Weekly Workout Plan 84
Weight Loss Weekly Workout Plan 90
Core Strenght & Flat Stomach Focus Weekly Workout Plan 96
30 Days Challenge 102

CHAPTER 6: NUTRITION AND WELL-BEING 111
NUTRITION TIPS FOR OPTIMAL PERFORMANCE IN WALL PILATES 111
MACRONUTRIENTS: 111
MICRONUTRIENTS AND THEIR SOURCES: 112
WEIGHT MANAGEMENT: WEIGHT LOSS, MAINTENANCE, AND MUSCLE GROWTH. 114

CONCLUSION 115

Introduction

What to Expect from This Book and why it's Unique and Effective:

In this comprehensive book, you're not just reading—you're embarking on a transformative fitness journey tailored specifically for Wall Pilates. What sets this guide apart? It's a multimedia experience complete with vivid images and step-by-step instructional videos that make each exercise crystal clear. Whether you're a beginner, intermediate, or advanced practitioner, you'll find meticulously designed workout programs for three different levels of expertise.

But that's not all! I've also included a 30-day challenge that will push you to new heights, ensuring you stay committed and see tangible results. These aren't just random exercises; these are targeted routines aimed at fulfilling specific fitness goals like weight loss, core strength, or flexibility.

And to round it all off, I offer nutritional advice and well-being tips to ensure a balanced, holistic approach to your health.

This guide is your ultimate resource for Wall Pilates, so why settle for less? Dive in and transform your fitness journey today!

Wall Pilates: The Essential You Need to Know

Wall Pilates, a contemporary offshoot of the classical Pilates method, has carved a niche for itself in the fitness world, evolving to meet the demands of modern practitioners. Its origins can be traced back to the innovative spirit of Joseph Pilates, who always emphasized adaptability and progression in his teachings. As enthusiasts sought ways to diversify their routines and adapt to space constraints, the wall emerged as an invaluable tool, offering both support and resistance. This adaptation not only made Pilates more accessible but also introduced a range of exercises that uniquely challenged the body's balance, strength, and flexibility.

There are several benefits of Wall Pilates. The wall's unyielding surface provides immediate feedback, ensuring that practitioners maintain optimal alignment and posture. Moreover, the added resistance when pushing or pulling against the wall amplifies muscle engagement, leading to enhanced strength and toning.

Furthermore, for those recovering from injuries or seeking a gentler introduction to Pilates, the wall offers the necessary support, allowing for a gradual progression in intensity.

We can say that the Wall Pilates exemplifies the evolution of fitness, demonstrating how traditional methods can be innovatively adapted to cater to contemporary needs while preserving their core principles.

Chapter 1: Wall Pilates: What You Really Need

Equipment and Tools

As you already know the Wall Pilates offers a unique blend of exercises that leverage the wall as a primary prop. To maximize the benefits of this practice and ensure safety, certain equipment and tools are recommended and in this chapter i will introduce you the essetial ones.

1. **Wall Unit**

The cornerstone of Wall Pilates, the wall unit, is a specialized piece of equipment designed to provide support, resistance, and versatility. Typically made of sturdy materials, it often features various attachments like springs, bars, and straps. These components allow for a wide range of exercises, targeting different muscle groups and offering varying levels of resistance.

Benefits:
- **Support:** The wall unit provides a stable anchor point, ensuring exercises are performed with proper alignment and form.
- **Versatility:** With its multiple attachments, the wall unit can be adapted for numerous exercises, catering to practitioners of all levels.
- **Safety:** Its robust construction ensures that exercises are done securely, minimizing the risk of injury.

2. **Pilates Mat**

While the wall is the primary focus in Wall Pilates, the floor plays a significant role in many exercises. A Pilates mat, thicker and denser than a regular yoga mat, is essential. It offers cushioning and support, especially for exercises that involve lying down or kneeling.

Benefits:
- **Comfort:** The mat provides a cushioned surface, protecting the spine, joints, and bones

during exercises.
- **Traction:** Made with non-slip materials, the Pilates mat ensures stability, preventing unwanted sliding or movement.
- **Hygiene:** A personal mat ensures cleanliness, especially when practicing in shared spaces.

3. Resistance Bands (Advised, Not Essential)

While not strictly necessary for Wall Pilates, resistance bands come highly recommended for those looking to intensify their workouts. These elastic bands offer varying degrees of resistance, allowing practitioners to customize the challenge level of their exercises.

Benefits:
- **Adaptability:** Available in different resistance levels, these bands cater to both beginners and advanced practitioners.
- **Enhanced Resistance:** For those seeking to amplify the challenge, resistance bands can add an extra layer of difficulty to exercises.
- **Portability:** Lightweight and compact, they are easy to carry, making them perfect for on-the-go workouts or travel.

Space Requirements & Practice Area

To reap the numerous benefits the wall pilates offers, it's crucial to have an appropriately set up practice area and in this paragraph i will give you some important info about the space requirements and i'll share with you essential considerations for creating an optimal Wall Pilates environment.

1. Assessing Space Requirements

it's essential to evaluate the space you have available. Here are some guidelines:

- **Wall Space:** Ideally, you'll need a clear wall area that's at least as tall as you and approximately 4 feet wide. This ensures you can perform a range of exercises without restriction.
- **Floor Space:** A clear area of about 6x6 feet in front of the wall will allow for adequate

movement, especially for exercises that require distance from the wall.
- **Ceiling Height:** Ensure there's enough overhead space, especially if you plan on incorporating jumping or standing exercises.

2. Choosing the Right Wall

Not all walls are created equal. Here's what to look for:

- **Sturdiness:** The wall should be solid and free from any signs of damage. Remember, you'll be leaning against it, so it needs to support your weight.
- **Free from Obstructions:** The chosen wall should be clear of any fixtures, decorations, or windows.
- **Smooth Surface:** A smooth wall is preferable as it reduces the risk of scratches or injuries.

3. Flooring Considerations

The floor is equally important in Wall Pilates. Here's what to consider:
Non-slip Surface: Hardwood, laminate, or a non-slip mat can be ideal. Avoid overly slippery surfaces to prevent accidents.
Cushioning: While you need stability, a bit of cushioning can be beneficial, especially for exercises that involve lying down. Consider using a thick Pilates or yoga mat.

4. Creating an Ambiance

Your Wall Pilates space should be inviting and conducive to concentration:

- **Lighting:** Natural light is ideal, but if that's not possible, opt for soft, ambient lighting.
- **Ventilation:** Ensure the room is well-ventilated. Fresh air can invigorate your practice.
- **Minimal Distractions:** Keep the space free from unnecessary clutter. Consider a dedicated space for Wall Pilates if possible.

Set Your Goals

In the same vein as traditional Pilates, having a roadmap for your wall Pilates regimen is essential for keeping you on track, energized, and aware of your progress. Here's a blueprint for effective planning:

Take Stock of Your Physical State: Before you begin, it's crucial to know your starting point. Consider:

- *How freely can you move your arms and legs?*
- *Are there any areas of discomfort or pain, such as in your back or joints?*
- *Is lying flat on your back comfortable for you?*
- *Do you have issues with maintaining balance?*
- *Do you need assistance for basic physical activities?*

These considerations will help you judge whether you're cut out for wall Pilates, which involves a variety of physical movements despite the added support of a wall.

Pinpoint What You Want to Accomplish: Clearly outline what you hope to gain from your wall Pilates sessions. It could be anything from enhancing your flexibility to strengthening your core.

Craft Real Objectives: Aim for goals that are:

Concrete: Instead of a broad aim like "get more flexible," specify what that means for you, such as being able to touch your toes.

Quantifiable: Have metrics in place to gauge your improvement.

Realistic: Choose goals that stretch you but are within your reach.

Aligned: Make sure your goals fit within your broader fitness aspirations and are suitable for wall Pilates.

Time-sensitive: Assign a timeframe to achieve your goals, adding a sense of urgency to your efforts.

Segment Your Goals: Split your overarching aim into smaller targets that serve as stepping stones toward your ultimate goal.

Formulate Your Strategy: Develop a well-defined routine that outlines how often and for how long you'll engage in wall Pilates each week.

Staying on Track and Fine-Tuning Your Approach: Consistency is the cornerstone of achieving your fitness objectives. However, it's equally important to be flexible with your regimen. For instance, if you experience discomfort while attempting certain stretches, consider slowing down or reducing the frequency for a while. You can revert to your original routine once you're back in form.

Tracking Your Journey: Keeping a record of your workouts is crucial for gauging your progress. Document the specific exercises, the number of sets and reps, and any adjustments you've made. Use these records in conjunction with your mini-goals to evaluate how far you've come.

Preparation Before Diving In: You've got your space set up and your goals outlined, but before you start your wall Pilates journey, there's more groundwork to be done. Understanding the fundamentals like proper alignment, posture, and core engagement is essential. This foundational knowledge not only enriches your exercise experience but also minimizes the risk of injury.

Chapter 2: Safety and Precautions

Like any physical activity, it comes with its set of risks and in this chapter i'll share with you the precautions you should take to ensure a safe and injury-free Wall Pilates experience.

1. Proper Alignment is Key

Understanding the importance of alignment is very important. Misalignment can lead to undue stress on joints and muscles, increasing the risk of injury.

Tip: Always start exercises with a neutral spine. Imagine a string pulling you up from the crown of your head, elongating your spine against the wall.

2. Warm-Up Before You Begin

Jumping straight into exercises can jolt cold muscles, making them prone to strains.

Tip: Dedicate at least 10 minutes to warming up. Gentle stretches and basic Pilates movements can prepare your body for more intensive wall exercises.

3. Know Your Limits

While pushing boundaries can lead to growth, it's essential to recognize and respect your body's limits. Overexertion can result in strains or even more severe injuries.

Tip: If a movement causes pain (not to be confused with discomfort), stop immediately. Consult a certified instructor to ensure you're performing the exercise correctly.

4. Use Proper Footwear

While traditional Pilates is often done barefoot, Wall Pilates may require more grip, especially when leveraging the wall for support.

Tip: Opt for non-slip socks or shoes with a good grip that are specifically designed for such workouts.

5. Ensure a Safe Environment

The wall you choose for your exercises should be sturdy and free from obstructions. Ensure there's enough space around you to move freely.

Tip: Remove any nearby furniture or potential tripping hazards. If using props, ensure they are in good condition and appropriate for the exercise.

6. Stay Hydrated

Muscles function best when they're well-hydrated. Dehydration can lead to muscle cramps and reduced performance.

Tip: Keep a water bottle nearby and take sips regularly, especially during longer sessions.

7. Focus on Breath

Breathing is a fundamental component of Pilates. Proper breath control can aid in movement precision and prevent unnecessary strain.

Tip: Typically, exhale on the effort of a movement and inhale on the release. This rhythm can help stabilize the core and provide more power to your exercises.

Remember: Maintaining concentration and awareness during these workouts is paramount. As practitioners glide, stretch, and push against the wall, the mind must be attuned to every subtle shift in the body. Distractions, both external and internal, can disrupt the flow and even lead to potential injuries.

To harness the full benefits of Wall Pilates, one must cultivate a deep sense of mindfulness. This involves being present in the moment, feeling each muscle contraction, and visualizing the body's movements in synchrony with the breath.

Such heightened awareness not only enhances the efficacy of each exercise but also transforms the workout into a meditative experience. Over time, this focused attention spills over into daily life, fostering a heightened sense of well-being and a deeper connection to one's physical self.

Chapter 3: Warm-Up and Cooldown

The Importance of Warm-Up

Just as a musician tunes their instrument before a performance, a Wall Pilates practitioner must prepare their body for the demands of the exercises ahead. Warm-up exercises serve to gradually elevate the heart rate, ensuring an efficient flow of oxygen-rich blood to the muscles.

This not only enhances flexibility but also reduces the risk of strains and injuries. The wall, a central component of this discipline, can be effectively utilized during warm-ups, providing tactile feedback and aiding in the alignment of the spine and limbs.

As one stretches and moves during the initial phase, the body becomes attuned to the wall, fostering a deeper connection and awareness.

This preparatory phase, often overlooked in haste, is the foundation upon which the success of a Wall Pilates session is built. It sets the tone, ensuring that the body and mind are synchronized, ready to embrace the challenges and reap the rewards of the workout.

Beyond Boosting Circulation, Warm-Ups Offer Additional Advantages:

Conditions the Joints: The initial exercises help to mobilize your joints, enhancing their flexibility and reducing the risk of injury or strain.

Engages Multiple Muscle Areas: By doing warm-ups, you're not just stretching but also activating a range of muscles, preparing them for the more intense workout to come.

Heightens Body Consciousness: These preliminary exercises also serve as a form of mindfulness, helping you become more aware of your body's alignment and movements, which is crucial when engaging in wall Pilates.

Readies the Core: Warm-ups also serve to activate your core muscles, like the transverse abdominis and pelvic floor, providing a strong foundation for the wall Pilates exercises to come.

Enhances Mental Focus: In addition to physical preparation, warm-ups help you mentally tune in, setting the stage for a focused and effective workout session.

WARM-UP EXERCISES

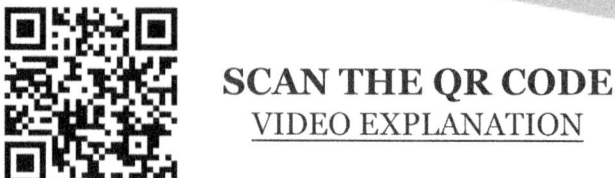

WALL MOUNTAIN CLIMBERS

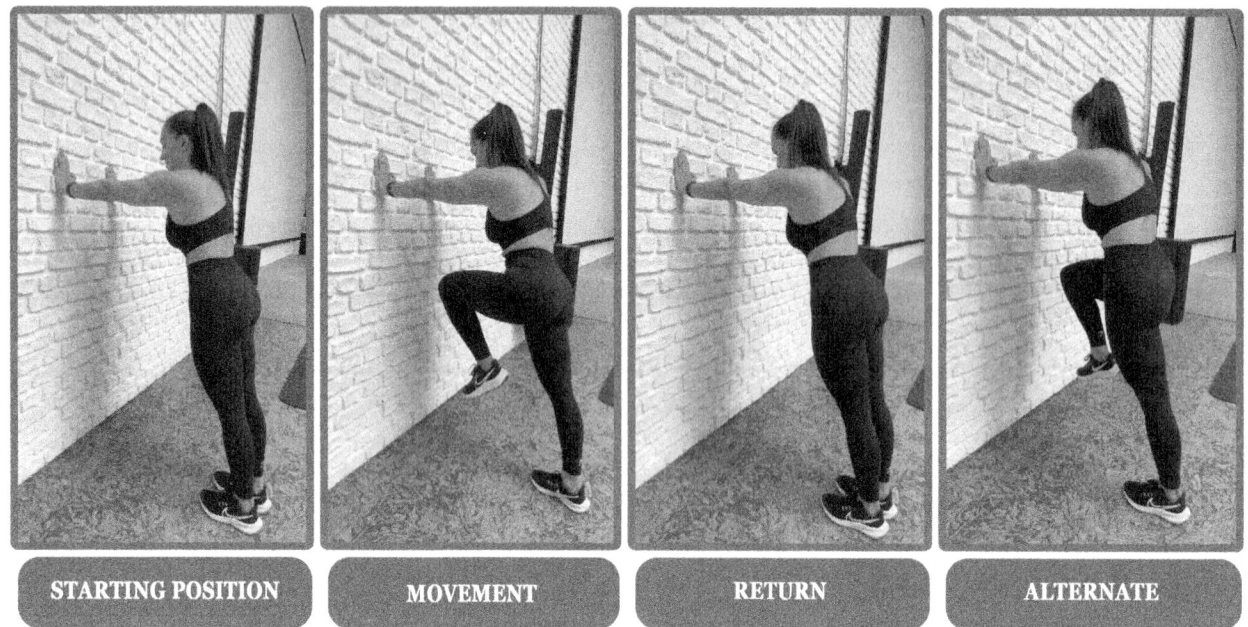

| STARTING POSITION | MOVEMENT | RETURN | ALTERNATE |

Starting Position: Begin by facing the wall. Place your hands on the wall at about chest height, slightly wider than shoulder-width apart. Walk your feet back and come into a plank position with your body at a slight angle to the wall. Ensure your core is engaged, and your body forms a straight line from head to heels.

Movement: Drive one knee towards your chest while keeping the rest of your body stable and your hips level. This mimics the climbing motion.

Return: Extend the leg back to its starting position.

Alternate: Repeat the movement with the other leg.

Continue: Perform the exercise for a set number of repetitions or time duration, alternating legs.

SCAN THE QR CODE
VIDEO EXPLANATION

WALL LATERAL LUNGES

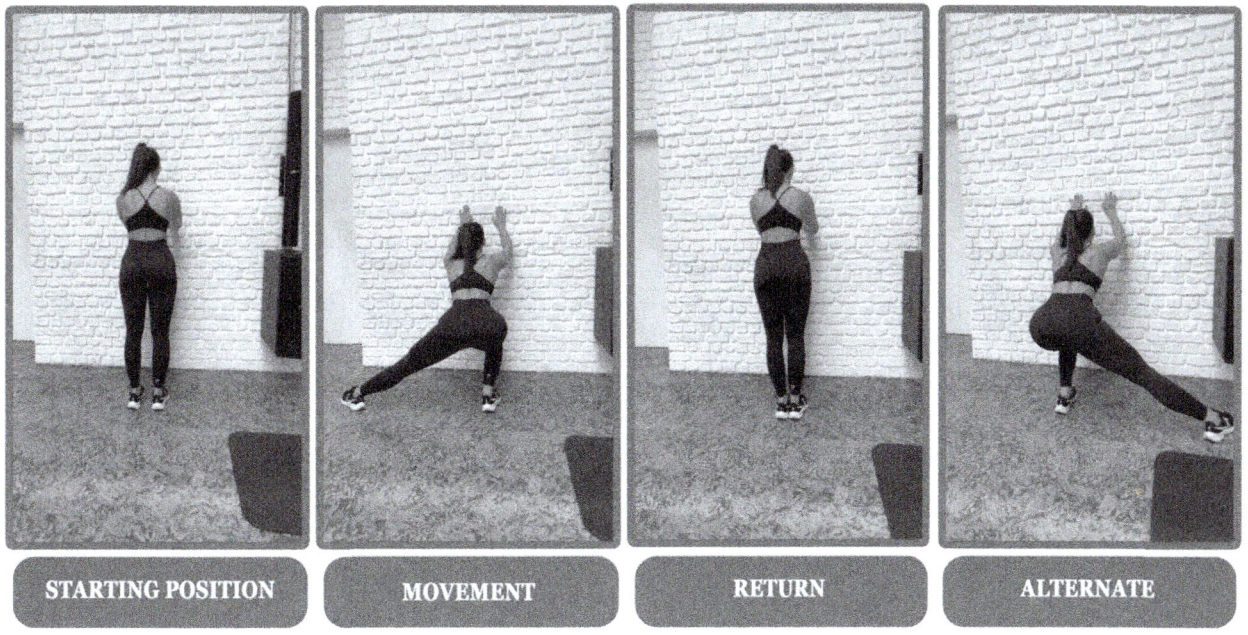

| STARTING POSITION | MOVEMENT | RETURN | ALTERNATE |

Starting Position: Stand facing the wall, with both arms resting against the wall for support.

Movement: Begin by extending one leg laterally (to the side), keeping it straight and parallel to the wall with the foot remaining on the ground. At the same time, the opposite leg stays close to the wall and bends forward, forming a 90° angle with the floor.

Wall Interaction: As you perform the movement, ensure that your arms remain in contact with the wall. This provides stability and ensures you are engaging your core and maintaining proper alignment. The wall serves as a guide and helps you maintain balance.

Return: Bring the extended leg and the bent one back to the starting position.

Alternate: repeat the movement with the other leg.

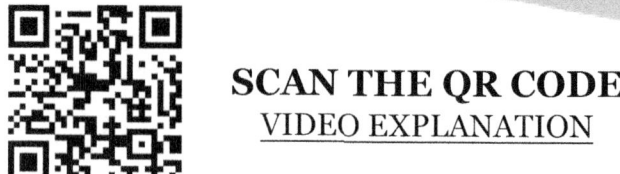

SCAN THE QR CODE
VIDEO EXPLANATION

WALL LEG SWINGS

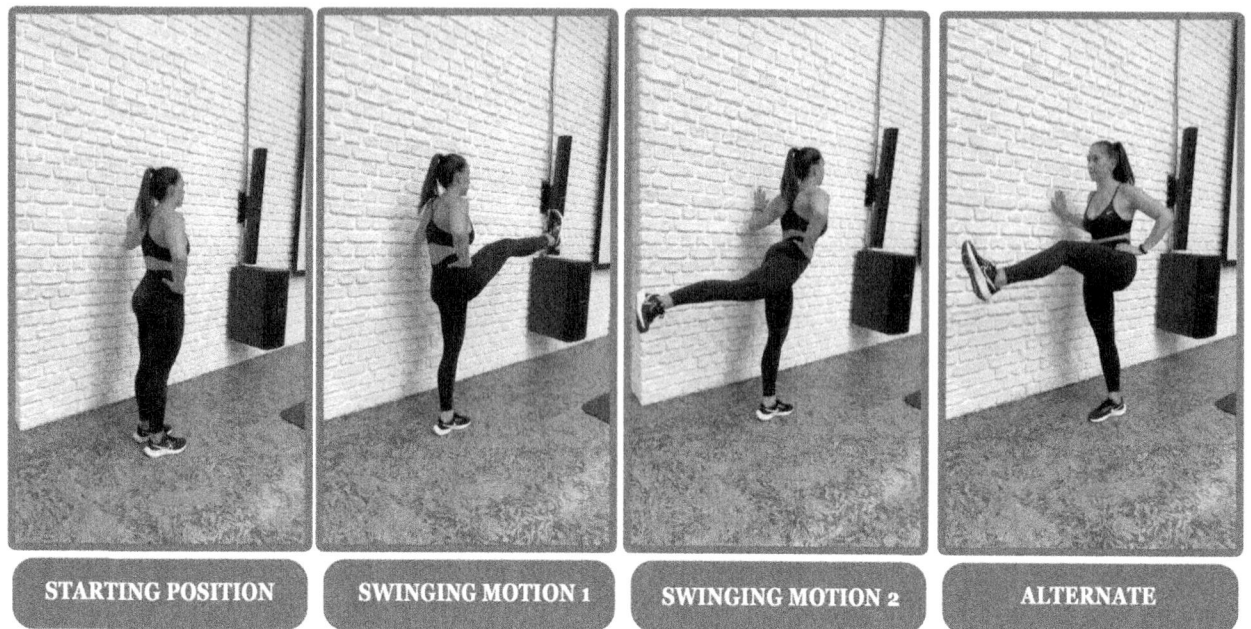

| STARTING POSITION | SWINGING MOTION 1 | SWINGING MOTION 2 | ALTERNATE |

Positioning: Stand sideways to the wall, with the side of your body near the wall. Extend your arm closest to the wall and rest it lightly against the wall with a slight bend at the elbow for support. Ensure you're standing at a comfortable distance from the wall to facilitate the swinging motion.

Starting Position: Shift your weight onto the leg closest to the wall.

Swinging Motion: Using the leg that is farther from the wall, swing it forward, raising it up in front of you to about hip height or as high as your flexibility allows. Then, swing it backward in a controlled motion as if delivering a kick behind you. Ensure you don't arch your back during the backward swing.

Switch: Repeat with the other side and repeat the movement.

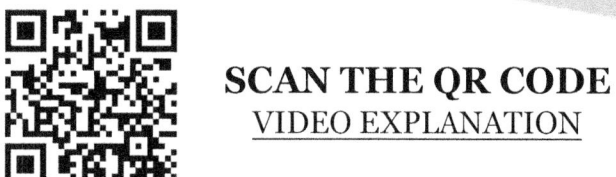

WALL SINGLE-LEG LIFTS

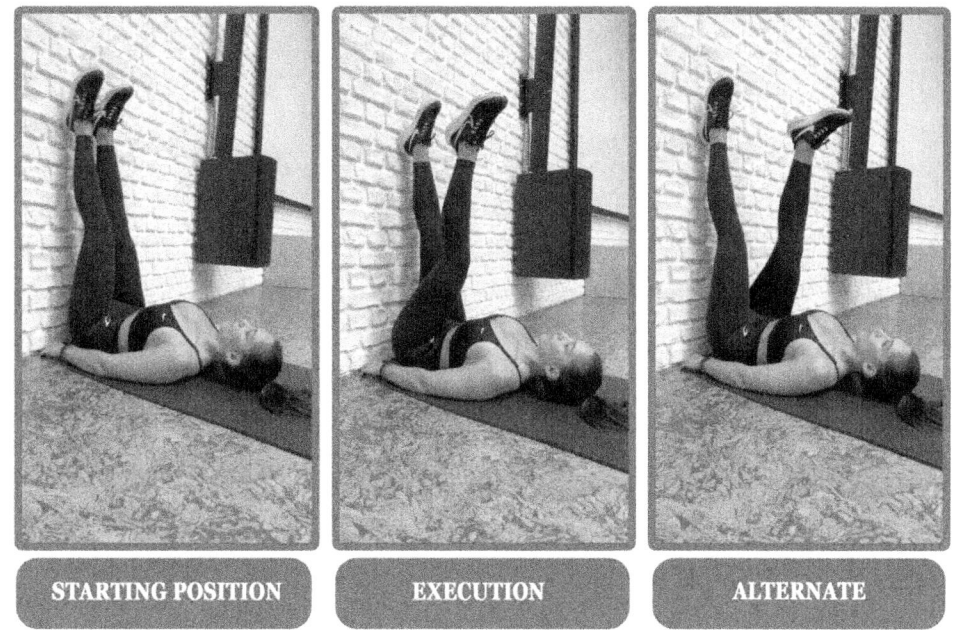

Position: Lie on your back on the ground, with your legs extended straight up against the wall. Your buttocks should be as close to the wall as possible, and your legs should be together.
Place your arms at your sides, palms facing down, for stability.

Execution: Engage your core muscles, pressing your lower back into the ground.
Slowly lower your right leg down towards the ground, keeping the knee straight. Go as far as you can without lifting your lower back off the ground.
Hold the lowered position for a moment, focusing on engaging the muscles in your core and leg.
Slowly lift the leg back up to meet the left leg against the wall.

Alternate: Repeat the movement with the left leg.

SCAN THE QR CODE
VIDEO EXPLANATION

WALL CALF RAISES

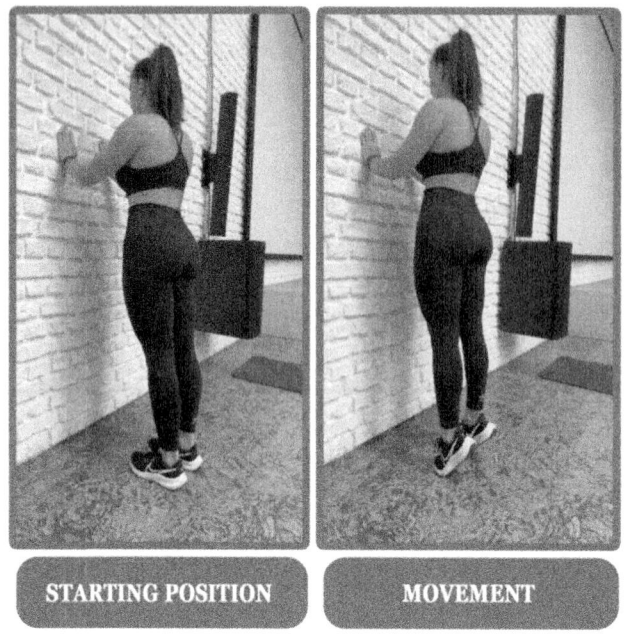

Position: Stand upright facing a wall with your feet hip-width apart. Place your hands on the wall at chest height for balance.

Movement: Slowly rise onto the balls of your feet, lifting your heels as high as possible to engage the calf muscles.
Hold the peak position for a moment, ensuring you're using your calf muscles and not pushing excessively with your hands.
Slowly lower your heels back to the ground.

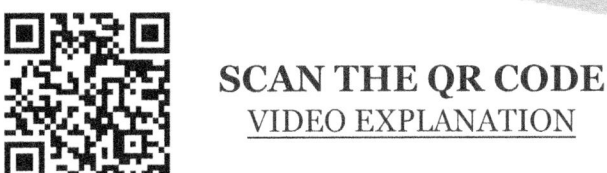

SCAN THE QR CODE
VIDEO EXPLANATION

ARM CIRCLES

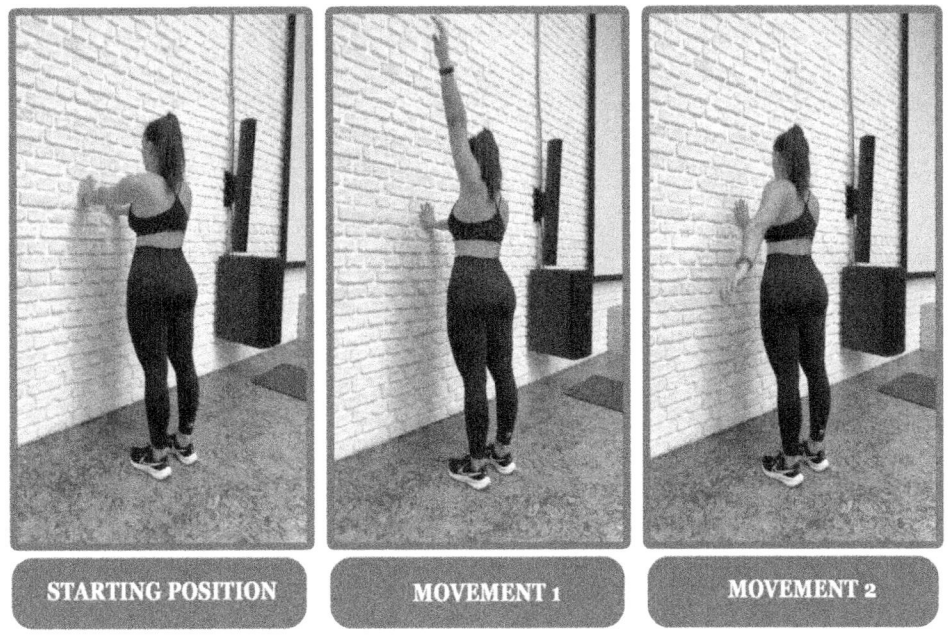

STARTING POSITION | MOVEMENT 1 | MOVEMENT 2

Positioning: Stand facing the wall, about an arm's length away. Your feet should be hip-width apart, and your posture should be upright.

Starting Position: Extend your arms forward so that your fingertips or palms (depending on arm length and comfort) are touching the wall at shoulder height.

Movement: Begin to make small circles with your arm, keeping the fingertips or palm in contact with the wall. The motion should originate from the shoulders. Ensure the movement is controlled and that you're not using momentum.

Alternate: Repeat with the other arm

Variations: You can perform the circles in both clockwise and counterclockwise directions. Over time, you can increase the size of the circles to challenge your shoulder mobility further. Another variation is to change the height of the hands, moving them higher or lower on the wall, to target different parts of the shoulder muscles.

SCAN THE QR CODE
VIDEO EXPLANATION

WALL SINGLE LEG CIRCLES

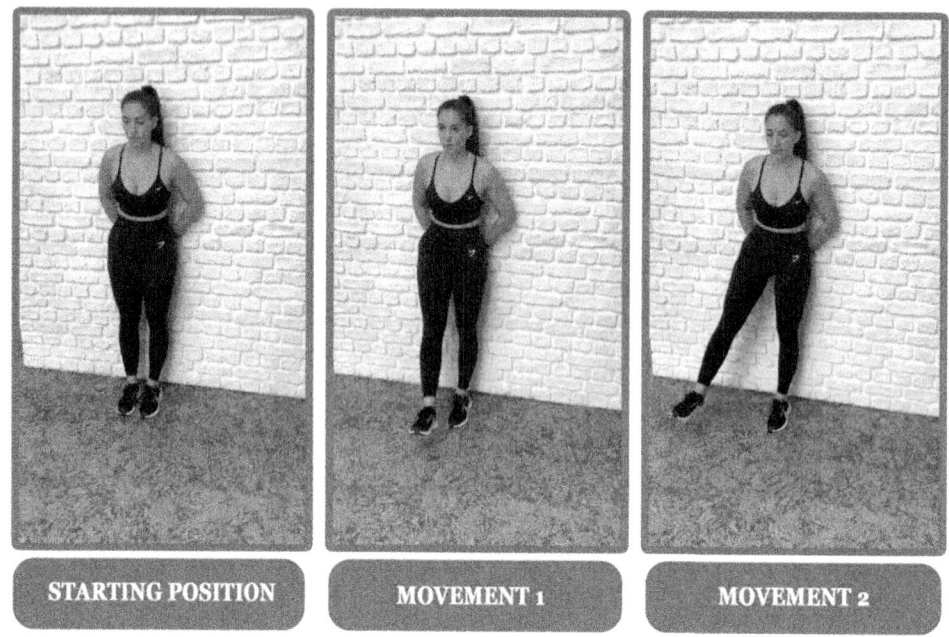

| STARTING POSITION | MOVEMENT 1 | MOVEMENT 2 |

Starting Position: Stand with your back against the wall, ensuring your head, shoulders, and hips are in contact with the wall.

Place your feet hip-width apart and about a foot away from the wall.

Engage your core muscles to press your lower back into the wall.

Execution: Slowly lift your right leg off the ground, keeping the knee straight or slightly bent based on your flexibility.

Begin to make controlled circles with your lifted leg. Ensure the movement originates from the hip joint and not the knee or ankle.

Keep your pelvis stable and avoid any tilting or shifting. The wall will provide feedback, ensuring you maintain a stable posture.

Alternate: Lower the leg back down and repeat with the left leg.

SCAN THE QR CODE
VIDEO EXPLANATION

WALL ANGELS

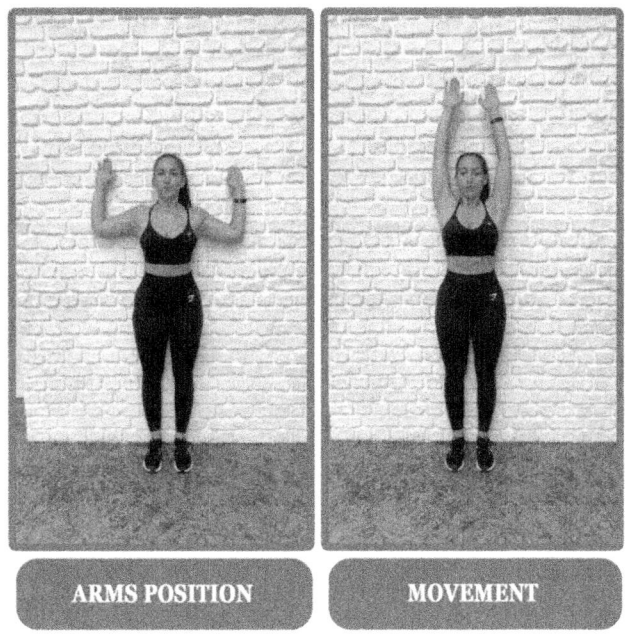

Starting Position: Stand with your back against a wall. Your feet can be a few inches away from the wall, and your knees should be slightly bent. The back of your head, upper back, and tailbone should be in contact with the wall.

Arms Position: Bend your elbows at a 90-degree angle and raise your arms to shoulder height, forming a "W" shape with your arms and torso. The backs of your hands, wrists, and elbows should be pressed against the wall as much as possible.

The Movement: Slowly slide your arms up the wall, trying to keep your wrists and elbows in contact with the wall. Extend them as high as you can without your back arching away from the wall. Your arms will form a "Y" shape at the top of the movement.

Return: Slowly slide your arms back down to the starting "W" position.

SCAN THE QR CODE
VIDEO EXPLANATION

KNEE TO NOSE

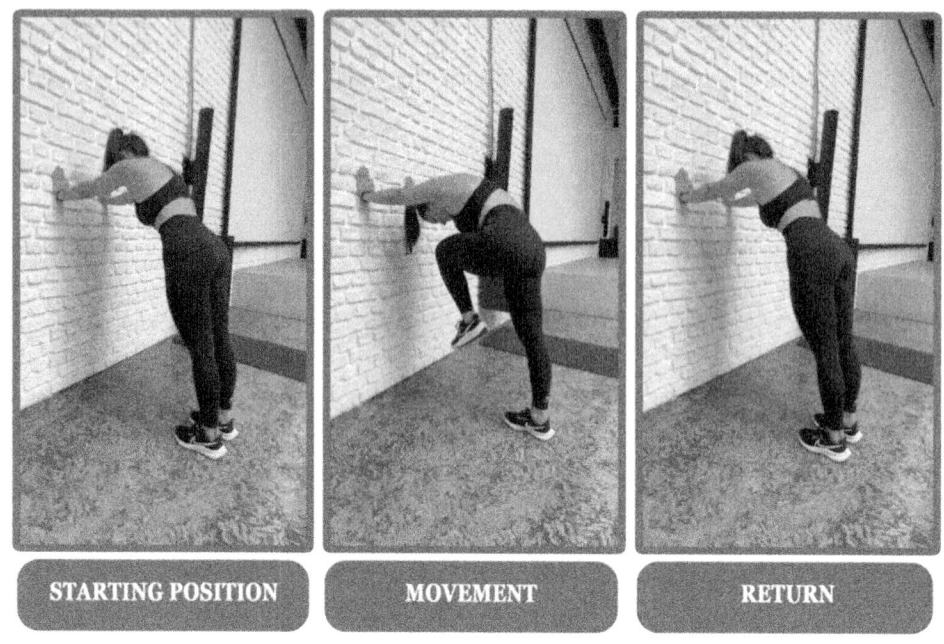

| STARTING POSITION | MOVEMENT | RETURN |

Starting Position: Stand facing the wall. Place your hands on the wall at shoulder height, fingers spread wide for stability. Step back a few feet so your body forms a diagonal line from head to heels.

Movement: Engage your core muscles. As you exhale, lift one knee towards your chest while simultaneously bringing your nose closer to the knee. Your spine will round slightly as you do this, and the foot of the moving leg will come off the ground.

Return: Inhale as you extend your leg back down to its starting position, pressing the ball of the foot into the ground and lengthening the spine to return to the diagonal line.

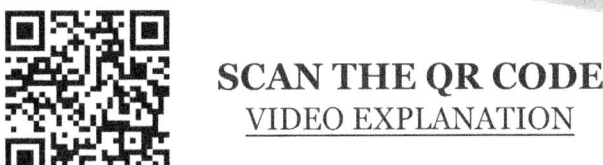

WALL LEG RAISE + KICK BACK

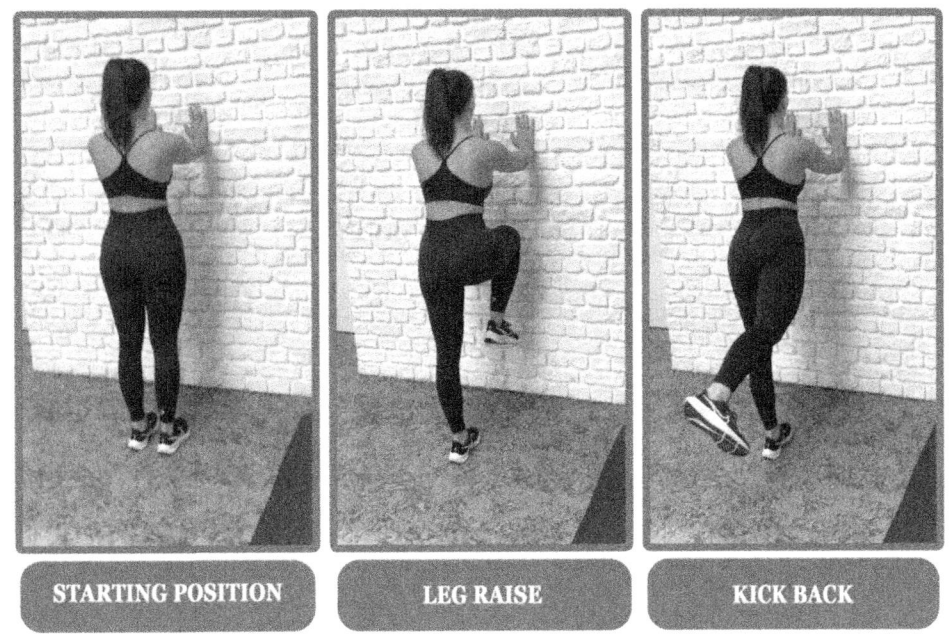

Starting Position: Stand facing the wall. Your arms are almost fully extended, with the palms of your hands resting against the wall, and your back is straight.

Leg Raise: Begin the exercise by lifting one knee up, as if you were delivering a knee strike. The knee should be at hip level or slightly higher. Engage your core to ensure stability.

Kick Back: From this position, extend the leg backward in a controlled kick. Keep your back straight and make sure to activate your glutes during this movement.

COOLDOWN EXERCISES

The Role of Cooldown Exercises

Cooldown exercises, often overshadowed by the intensity of core Wall Pilates movements, play a pivotal role in the holistic approach to this unique fitness regimen. These exercises serve as a bridge, transitioning the body from a state of heightened activity to a state of rest, ensuring that the muscles, heart rate, and breathing gradually return to their baseline levels.

In the context of Wall Pilates, cooldown techniques often involve gentle stretches and controlled breathing exercises performed against the wall. For instance, a wall-assisted hamstring stretch not only elongates the muscles worked during the session but also provides feedback on alignment and posture.

Similarly, deep wall slides, where one slides down the wall into a seated position while taking deep breaths, can help in releasing tension from the back and hips.

Incorporating these cooldown techniques not only minimizes the risk of injury and muscle soreness but also enhances flexibility and promotes mental relaxation. As practitioners conclude their Wall Pilates session, it's this phase of deliberate and mindful cooling down that ensures they carry the benefits of their workout into their daily lives, feeling both physically rejuvenated and mentally centered.

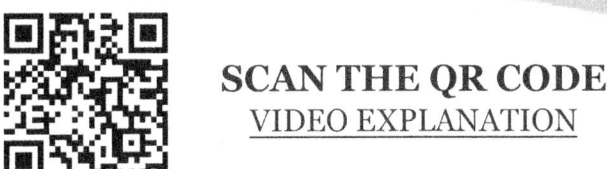

WALL COBRA POSE

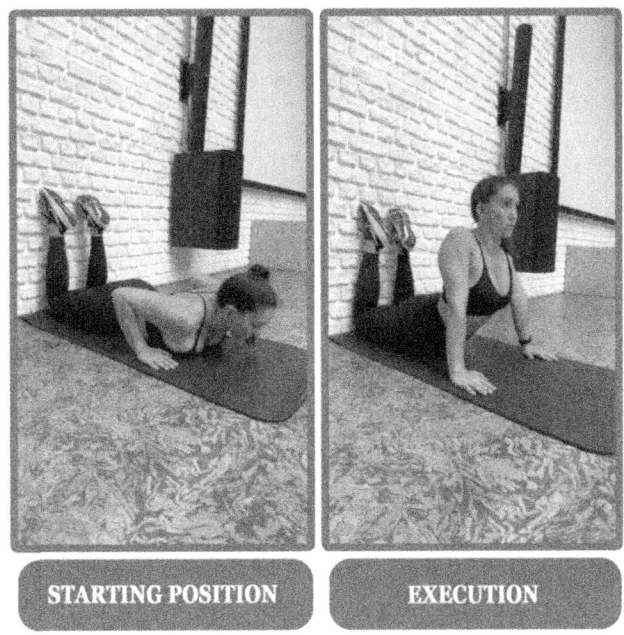

Starting Position: Start by lying face down with your shins and feet pressed against the wall and your thighs on the mat, forming a 90° angle with your legs. Your arms are positioned laterally as if you're about to do a push-up.

Execution: Use the strength of your arms and shoulders to lift yourself up, keeping your feet and shins pressed against the wall. Engage your core to ensure stability.

Hold and Return: Once lifted, hold this position for a moment, ensuring you have a correct posture and are activating the appropriate muscles. Slowly lower your body, returning to the initial position with your thighs on the mat.

Purpose: This stretch targets the chest, shoulders, and front of the torso. It's excellent for counteracting the forward hunch that many of us develop from sitting at desks or looking down at our phones. The wall provides support, allowing you to control the depth of the stretch and ensuring proper alignment.

SCAN THE QR CODE
VIDEO EXPLANATION

WALL CAT POSE

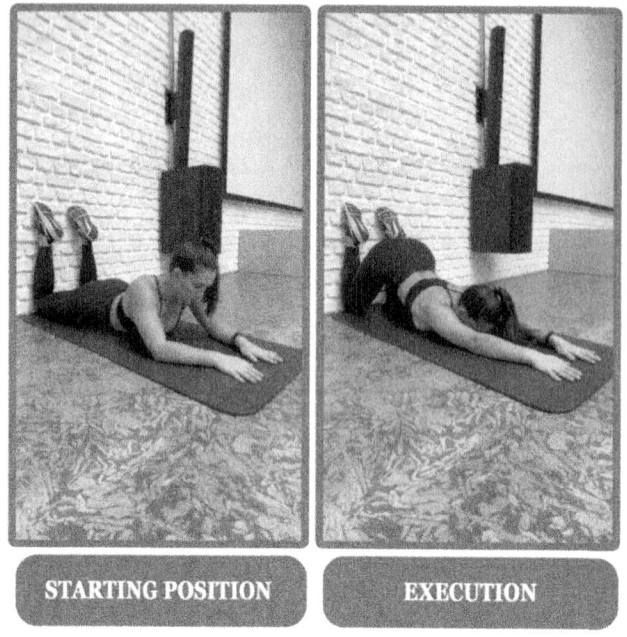

Starting Position: Start by lying face-down on your mat, propped up on your elbows which are bent at a 90-degree angle and positioned in front of you. Your knees should be leaning against the wall, and your shins pressed to it.

Execution: From here, extend your arms to straighten them, pushing your hips back until they meet your heels. Return to your initial position. Coordinate your breathing by exhaling as you lift your hips and inhaling as you come back down to your elbows.

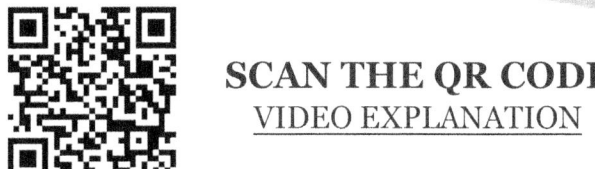

LOWER BODY STRETCH

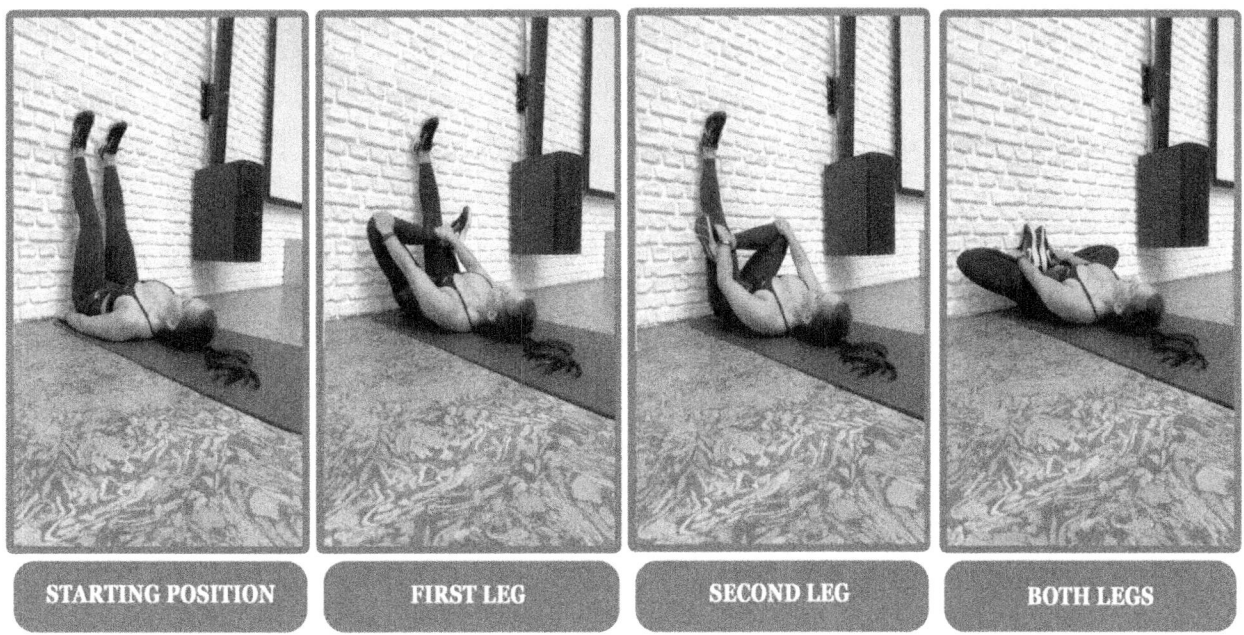

Positioning: Begin by lying on your back on the floor, close to a wall. Your buttocks should be as close to the wall as comfortably possible, with your legs extended straight up the wall.

Into the Stretch: Slowly open your legs in a "V" shape, allowing gravity to pull them down towards the floor. This will stretch the inner thighs.

Outer Hip Stretch: For a deeper stretch into the outer hips and glutes, bend your knees and place your feet together on the wall, allowing your knees to drop out to the sides.
This position resembles a butterfly stretch but is assisted by the wall.
You can deepen the stretch by gently pressing on your thighs or knees, pushing them closer to the floor. Ensure you do this gently and without forcing the stretch.

Release: To come out of the stretch, use your hands to support your legs as you bring them back together and up the wall. Slowly roll to one side and use your arms to push yourself up to a seated position.

SCAN THE QR CODE
VIDEO EXPLANATION

WALL-ASSISTED PUPPY POSE

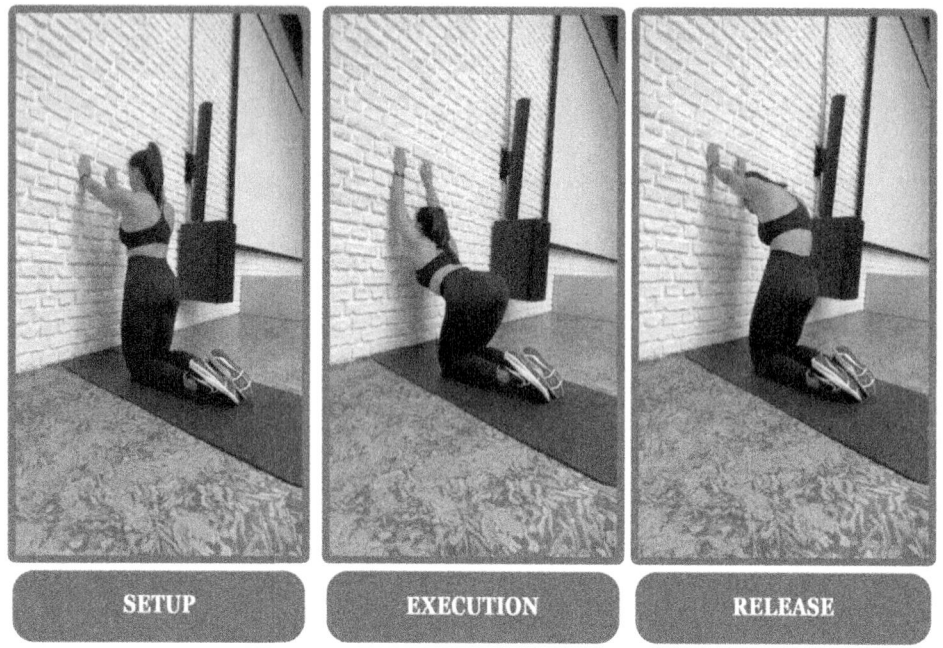

SETUP　　　　　EXECUTION　　　　　RELEASE

Starting Position: Begin by facing the wall. Stand a couple of feet away from it.

Setup: Place your hands on the wall at about chest height, fingers spread wide.

Execution: As you exhale, begin to walk your feet back and bend at the hips, allowing your chest to move towards the floor. Your arms should remain straight, and your hands pressed against the wall. The aim is to create a stretch along the spine and in the shoulders.

Deepening the Stretch: To deepen the stretch, you can walk your hands further up the wall or step your feet further back. Ensure that your hips remain above your knees.

Hold: Maintain the pose for several breaths, feeling the stretch in your shoulders, chest, and spine.

Release: To come out of the pose, walk your feet forward and slowly lift your torso, returning to the starting position.

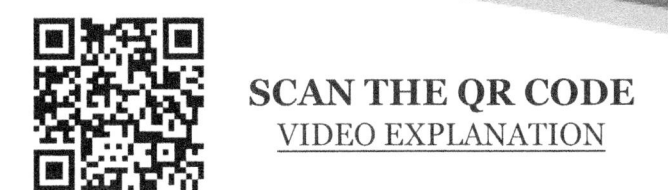

WALL SPHINX POSE

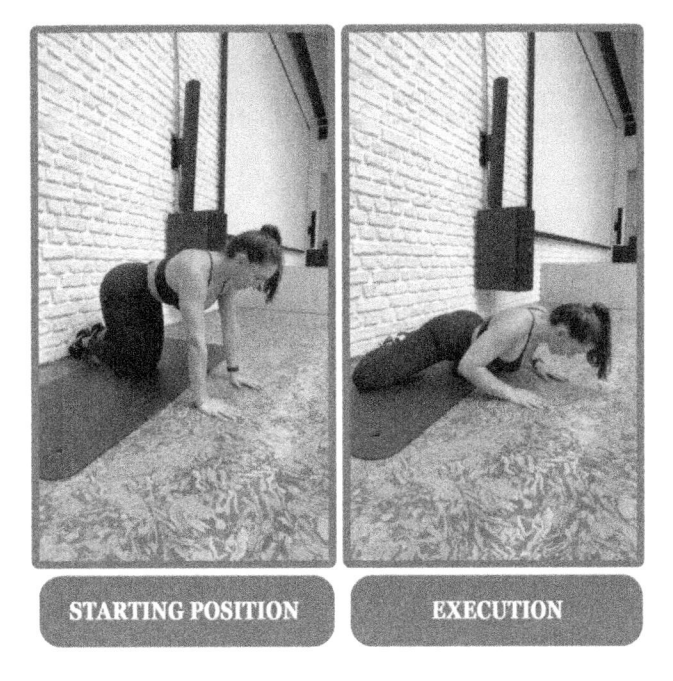

Starting Position: Start by laying face down, positioning your feet against a wall.

Execution: Elevate yourself onto your forearms, making sure your elbows are directly beneath your shoulders. Push down into the floor with your palms and forearms to lift your chest, creating a gentle arch in your back. Intensify the stretch by pressing your feet into the wall.

Chapter 4: Comprehensive Wall Pilates Exercises

ABS & CORE EXERCISES

SCAN THE QR CODE
VIDEO EXPLANATION

ABS AND CORE CRUNCH VERSION

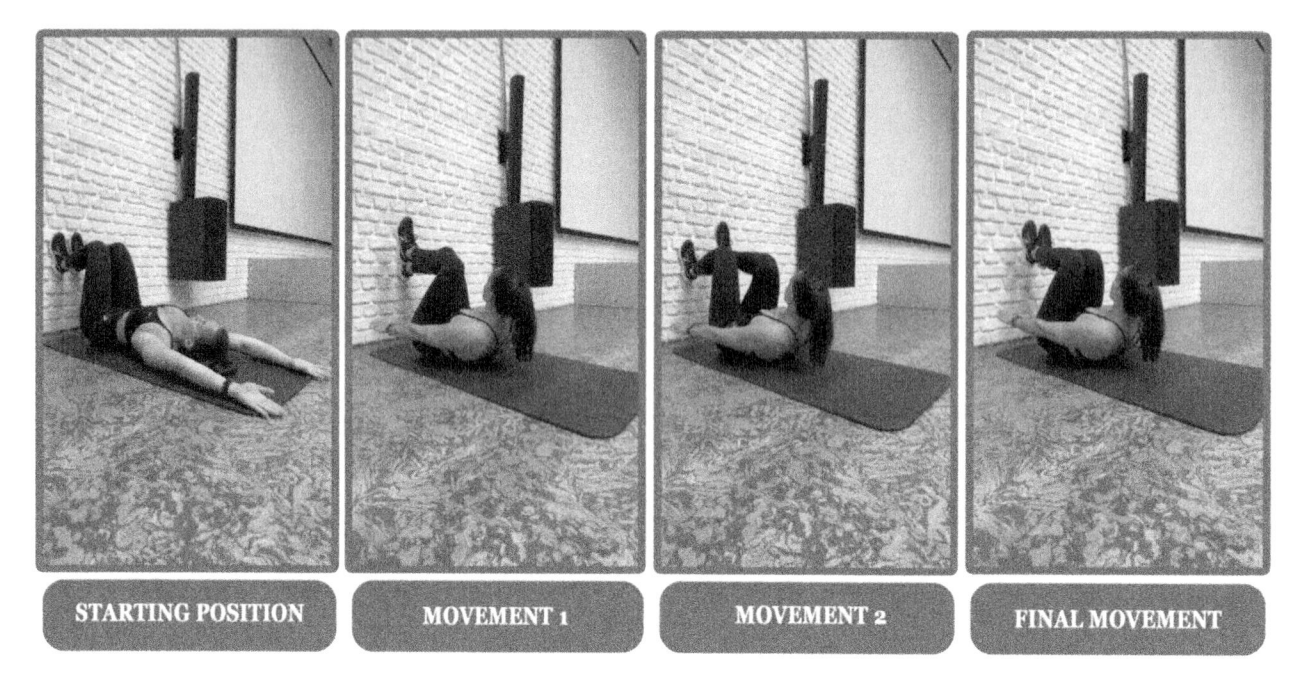

| STARTING POSITION | MOVEMENT 1 | MOVEMENT 2 | FINAL MOVEMENT |

Starting Position: Start by lying flat on the floor with your back pressed against it. Your knees should be bent, and your feet should be resting against the wall. Extend your arms above your legs, as depicted in the illustration.

Movement 1: Raise your upper body and draw your right knee close to your head. Keep your arms at your sides to help you balance and maintain proper form. Maintain this pose for a count of three.
Go back to your initial lying position.

Movement 2: Next, elevate your upper body and bring your left knee towards your head. Your arms should be at your sides again. Hold this for three seconds.
Revert to the starting position.

Final Movement: Finally, lift your torso and draw both knees towards your head. Keep your arms at your sides to help you balance. Hold this for another three seconds.
Return to your original lying position to complete the exercise.

SCAN THE QR CODE
VIDEO EXPLANATION

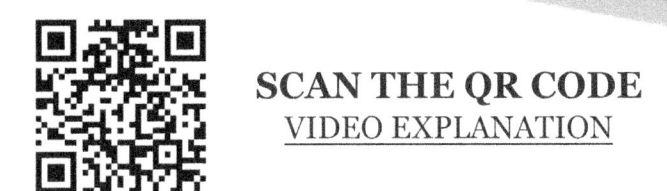

ABS AND CORE OBLIQUE VERSION

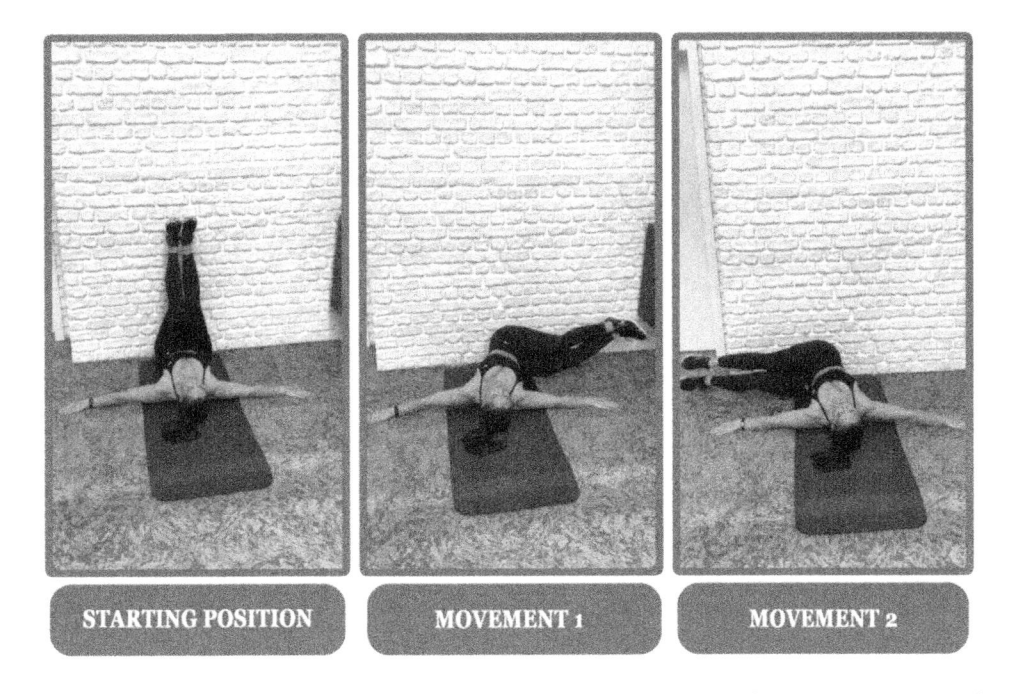

| STARTING POSITION | MOVEMENT 1 | MOVEMENT 2 |

Starting Position: Start by lying flat on the floor, with your back touching it and your legs and buttocks against a wall. Extend your arms to your sides, palms facing up.

Movement 1: Shift your legs to the right while keeping your arms stationary and your back flat on the floor. Pause for a moment in this position. Then, revert to your initial posture.

Movement 2: Next, swing your legs to the left, holding briefly. Your legs should mimic the back-and-forth motion of windshield wipers on a car. Finally, come back to the starting position.

SCAN THE QR CODE
VIDEO EXPLANATION

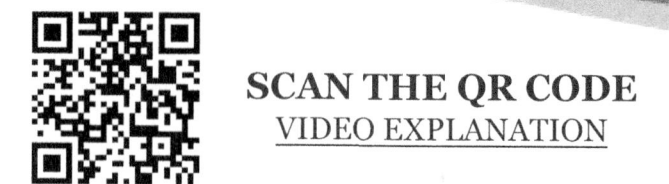

WALL BICYCLE CRUNCHES

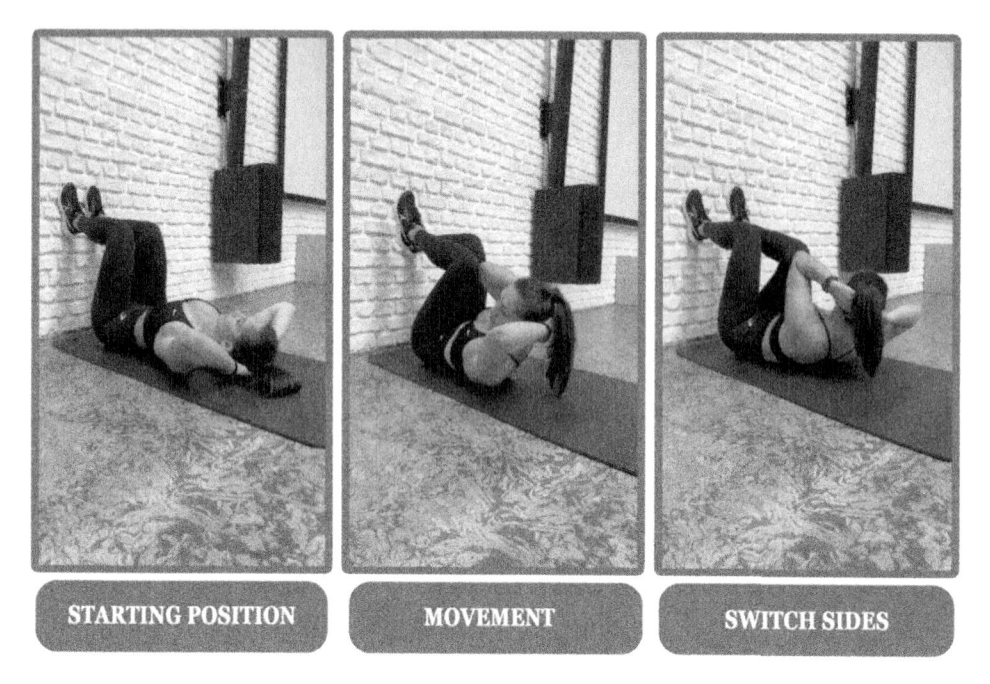

STARTING POSITION | **MOVEMENT** | **SWITCH SIDES**

Positioning: Start by lying on your back on a mat, with your hips close to the wall. Place your legs up against the wall, with your knees bent at a 90-degree angle.

Engage Core: Press your lower back into the mat, engaging your core muscles. Place your hands behind your head, elbows wide.

Movement: Begin by bringing your right elbow towards your left knee while extending your right leg straight out, keeping it elevated a few inches off the ground. Ensure your leg remains parallel to the floor.

Switch Sides: Return to the starting position and then bring your left elbow towards your right knee while extending your left leg.

WALL PIKE CRUNCHES

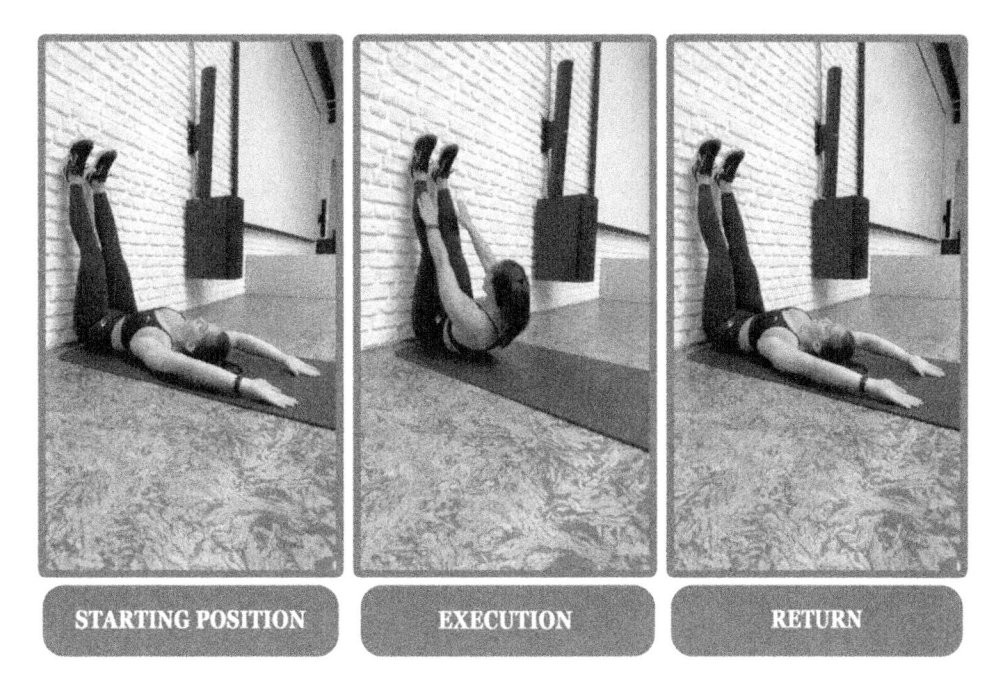

STARTING POSITION | **EXECUTION** | **RETURN**

Starting Position: Begin by lying down on a mat, ensuring your lower back is flush against the wall (refer to the diagram for clarity).
Elevate your legs and keep them close together against the wall. Place your hands flat on the ground, positioned behind your head.

Execution: Aim to reach your ankles with outstretched arms while maintaining your feet's position on the wall. Subsequently, revert to your initial pose.

Return: Coordinate your breathing by exhaling as you lift yourself and inhaling as you descend back onto the mat.

SCAN THE QR CODE
VIDEO EXPLANATION

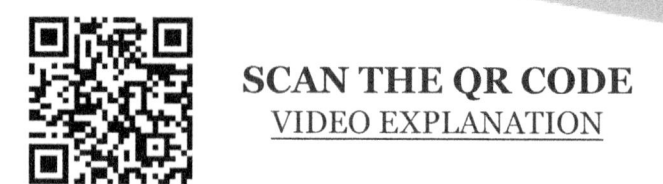

WALL ABDOMINAL PRESS LEGS VERSION

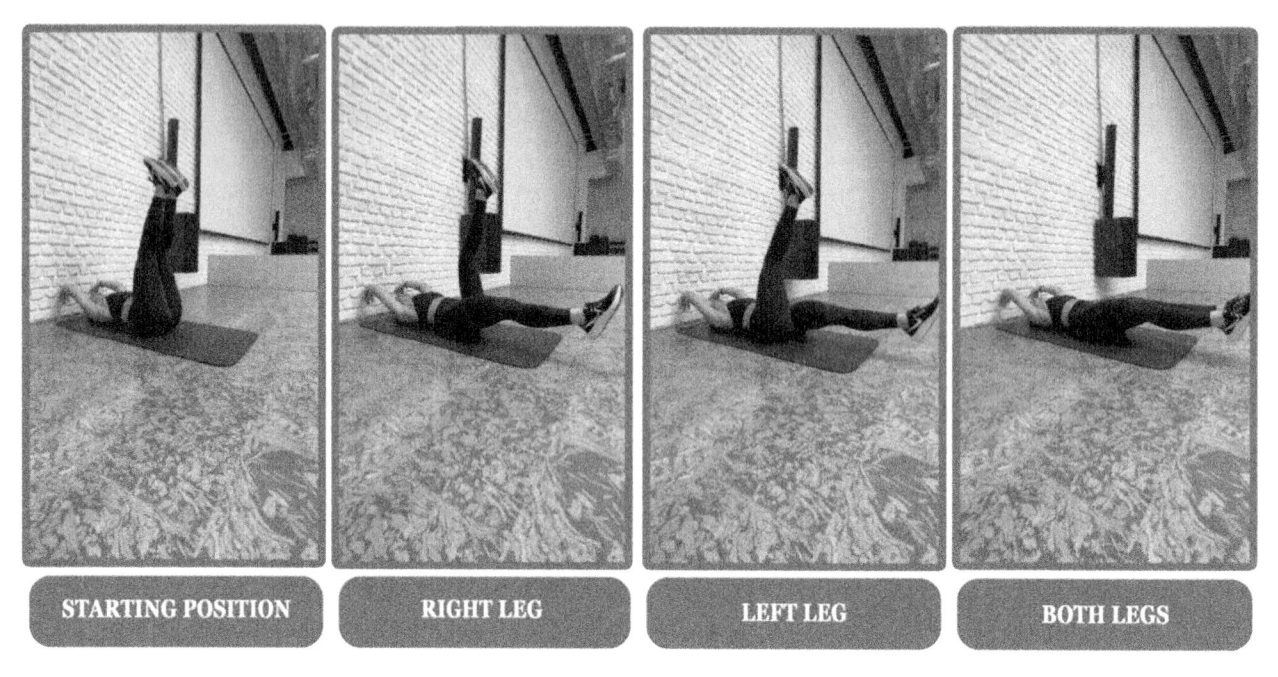

| STARTING POSITION | RIGHT LEG | LEFT LEG | BOTH LEGS |

Starting Position: Begin by lying on your back, hands pressed against the wall above your head, and legs elevated straight up. First, engage your core muscles.

Right Leg: Then, in a controlled manner, lower your right leg towards the floor without actually touching it, and bring it back up.

Left Leg: Next, do the same with your left leg.

Both Legs: Finally, lower both legs in a similar fashion and return them to the starting position.

Remember to breathe out as you lower your legs and breathe in as you lift them back up.

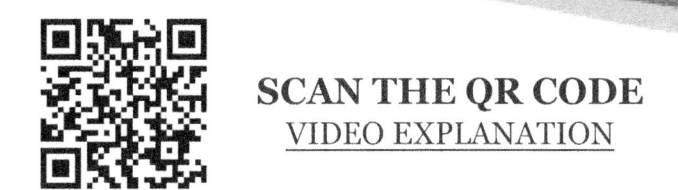

SUPERMAN

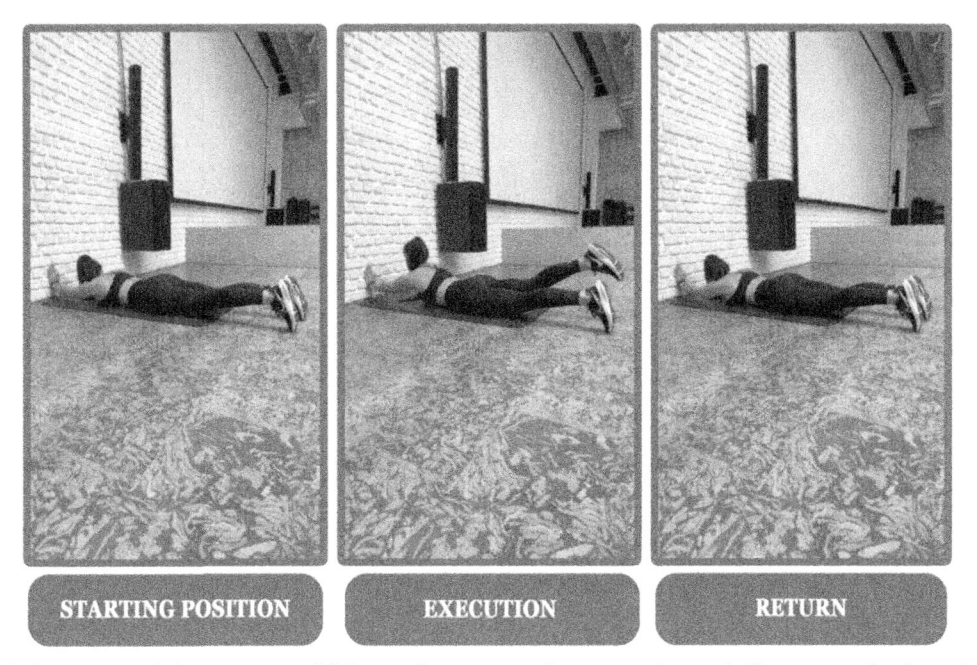

STARTING POSITION | **EXECUTION** | **RETURN**

Starting Position: Position yourself face-down on the mat, legs fully extended and toes pointing outward.

Execution: Extend your right arm in front of you, elbow bent, as shown in the diagram. Use your left hand for wall support. On an exhale, elevate your right leg, leading with your toe tips and keeping the knee straight.

Return: Inhale as you bring the leg back down.

Switch sides, raising your left leg while using your right hand for wall support.

SCAN THE QR CODE
VIDEO EXPLANATION

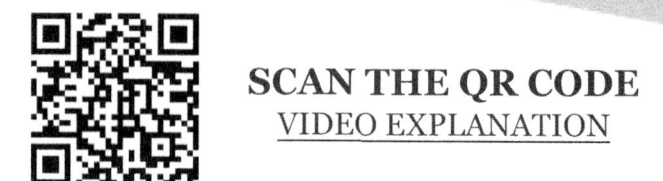

WALL TEASER ABS CORE

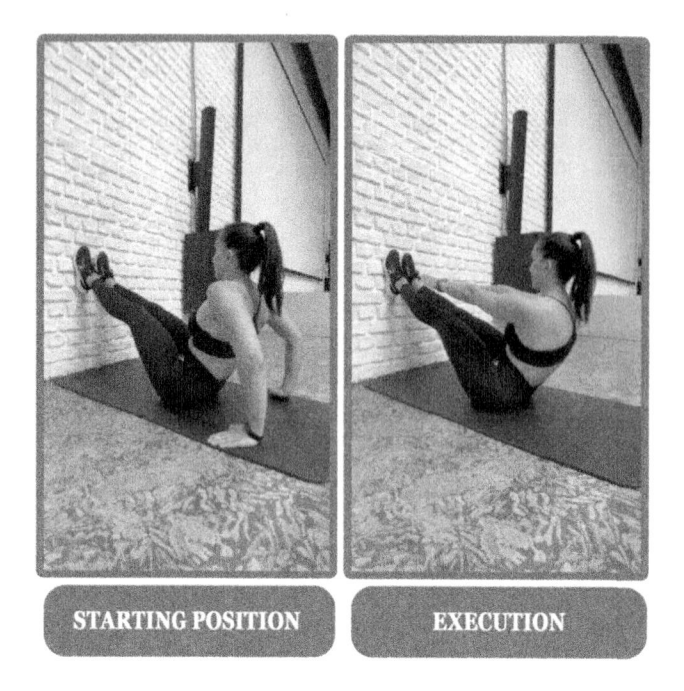

STARTING POSITION   **EXECUTION**

Starting Position: Begin by sitting on the floor with your legs extended in front of you and your heels pressed against the wall. Your back should be upright, and your arms extended forward at shoulder height.

Engage the Core: Inhale deeply, and as you exhale, engage your core muscles by drawing your navel towards your spine.

Achieve the Teaser Position: Continue to roll down until you're in a C-curve position with your lower back on the floor, your upper back and shoulders lifted, and your legs lifted at a 45-degree angle against the wall. Your arms should remain extended forward, parallel to your lifted legs.

Hold and Return: Hold the Teaser position for a breath, feeling the engagement in your core. Exhale and slowly roll your spine back up to the starting position, sliding your feet down the wall.

SCAN THE QR CODE
VIDEO EXPLANATION

WALL WALKING PLANK

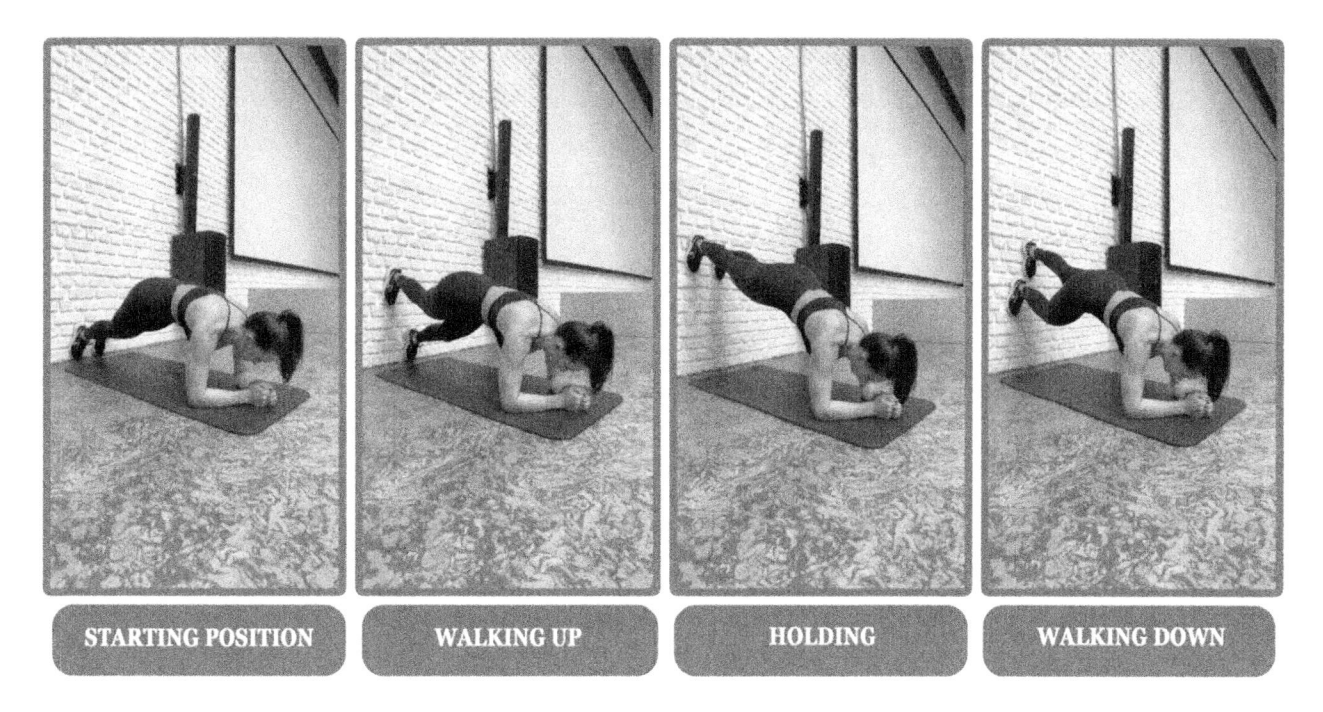

STARTING POSITION | **WALKING UP** | **HOLDING** | **WALKING DOWN**

Starting Position: Begin in a traditional plank position with your forearms resting on the ground, elbows aligned under your shoulders, and your feet close to the wall.

Walking Up: Pushing through your hands, start "walking" your feet up the wall. As you do this, your body will move closer to the wall. It's essential to keep the core engaged and maintain a straight line from your hands to your feet. Go as high as you feel comfortable.

Holding the Position: Once you've walked your feet up to your desired height, hold the position. Ensure your hands are shoulder-width apart, your core is tight, and your shoulders are engaged.

Walking Down: Carefully start "walking" your feet back down the wall, returning to the starting plank position. It's crucial to control this movement and not rush, as controlling the descent is where a lot of the strength-building comes into play.

SCAN THE QR CODE
VIDEO EXPLANATION

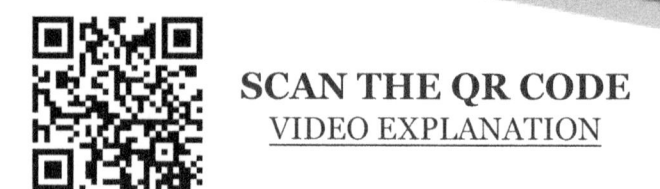

DOLPHINE POSE

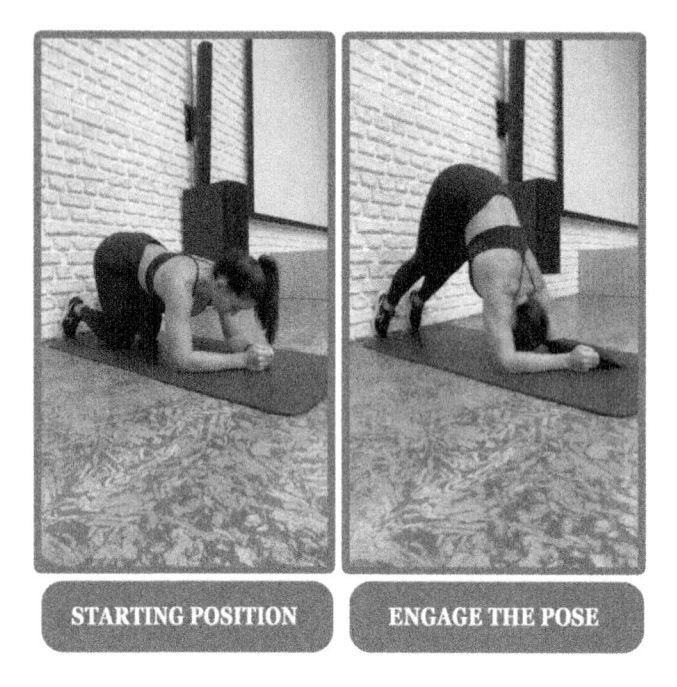

STARTING POSITION **ENGAGE THE POSE**

Starting Position: Begin by facing the wall. Place your forearms on the ground, ensuring they are shoulder-width apart. Your elbows should be directly below your shoulders. Extend your legs behind you, with your feet hip-width apart.

Engage the Pose: Tuck your toes under and lift your hips towards the ceiling, coming into an inverted "V" shape. Your body should resemble a downward-facing dog, but on your forearms.

Wall Support: For those new to the pose or seeking additional stability, press the heels gently into the wall. This provides stability, allows for a deeper stretch, and ensures the hips are lifted high, emphasizing the elongation of the spine.

Hold and Breathe: Engage your core, press your forearms into the ground, and keep your neck neutral. Breathe deeply and hold the pose for several breaths.

Release: To come out of the pose, gently lower your knees to the ground and rest in a child's pose.

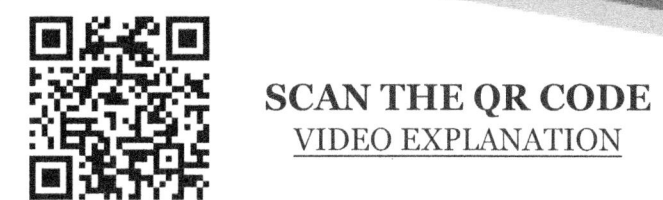

DOLPHINE POSE WITH FEET ELEVATED ON WALL

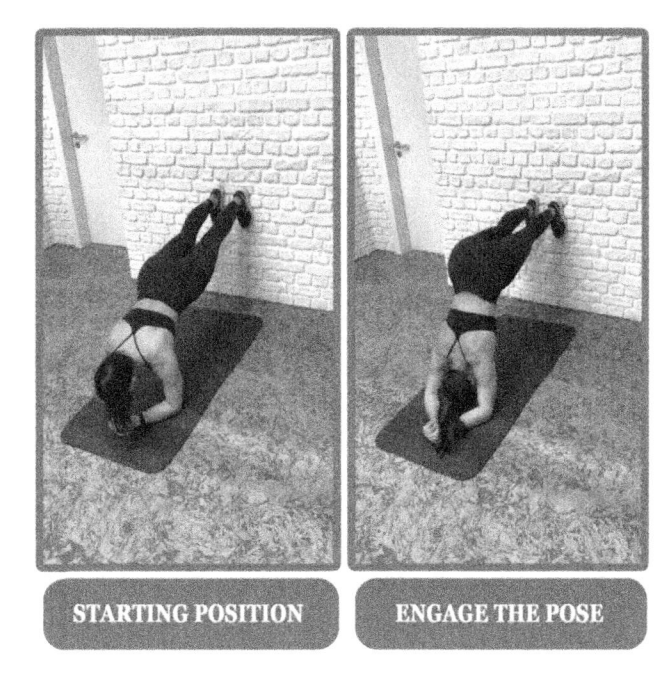

Starting Position: Begin by facing away from the wall. Place your forearms on the ground, ensuring they are shoulder-width apart. Your elbows should be directly below your shoulders. Walk your feet up the wall so that they are elevated, with your body forming an angle. The exact height of the feet on the wall can vary based on flexibility and comfort.

Engage the Pose: Press down firmly through your forearms and lift your hips up and back, aiming to create an inverted "V" shape with your body. The elevation of the feet intensifies the pose, adding an element of inversion.

Alignment: Ensure your head is positioned between your upper arms and is not hanging down or overly lifted. Engage your core muscles to support the spine and maintain balance.

Hold, Breathe and Release: Breathe deeply, drawing attention to the stretch in the hamstrings and calves. The elevation of the feet also brings a deeper engagement to the shoulders and upper back. Hold the pose for several breaths, or as long as it's comfortable. To come out of the pose, carefully walk your feet down the wall and lower your knees to the ground.

SCAN THE QR CODE
VIDEO EXPLANATION

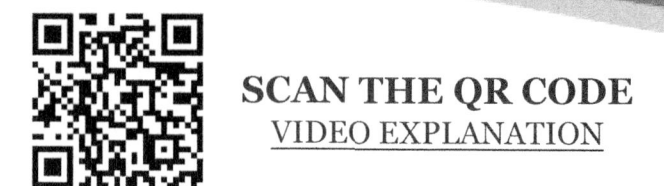

REVERSE CURL

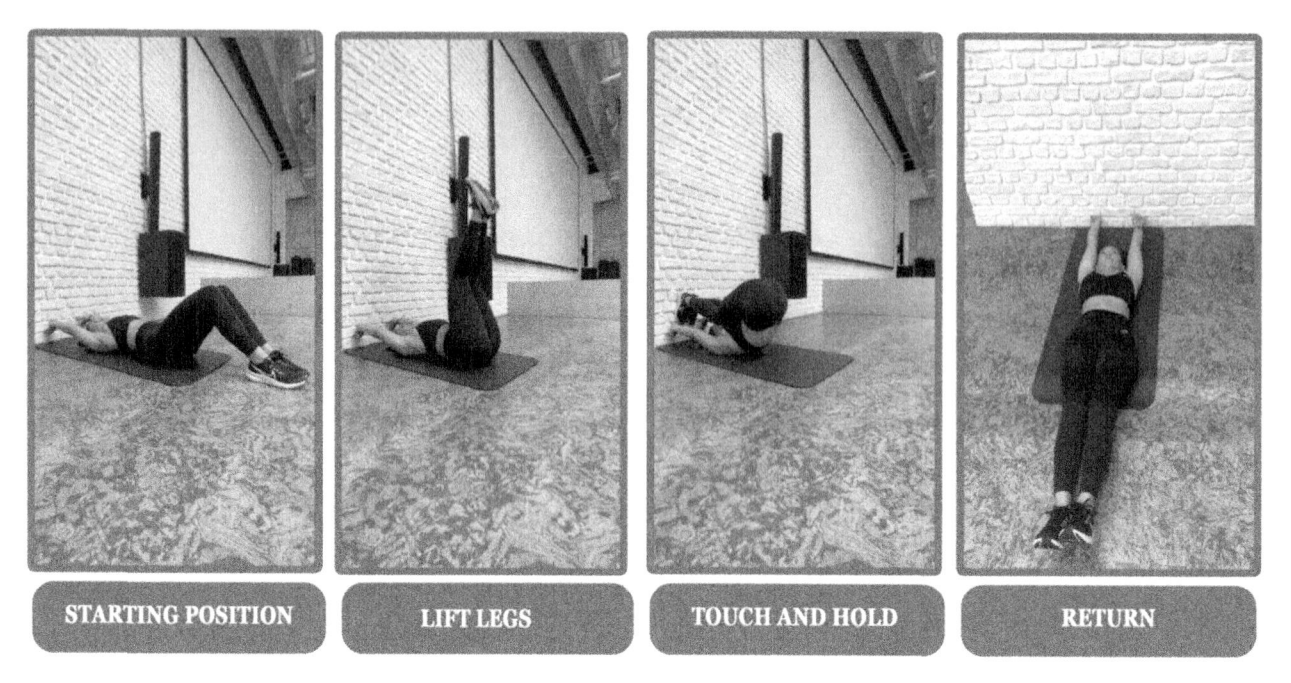

| STARTING POSITION | LIFT LEGS | TOUCH AND HOLD | RETURN |

Position: Stand facing away from the wall, about a foot or two away. Place your hands on the wall behind you at shoulder height.

Engage Core: Engage your core muscles and maintain a neutral spine.

Lift Legs: Slowly lift your legs, bending your knees and bringing your feet toward your hands on the wall.

Touch and Hold: Try to touch your feet to your hands or get as close as possible, holding the position for a few seconds. This will require strong core engagement and balance.

Return: Slowly lower your legs back down to the starting position.

ARMS & SHOULDERS STRETCHES AND STRENGHTING EXERCISES

SCAN THE QR CODE
VIDEO EXPLANATION

ARM BENDS

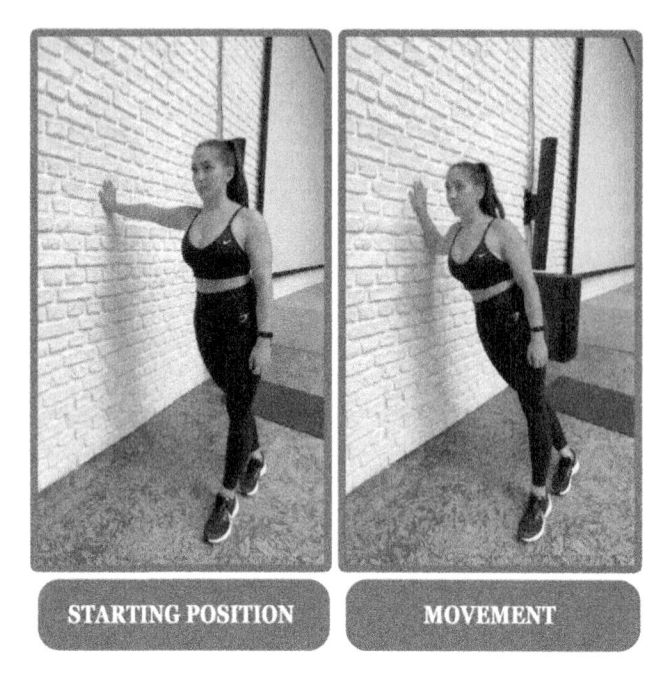

STARTING POSITION | **MOVEMENT**

Starting Position: Stand sideways to the wall, about an arm's length away.
Place your palm flat against the wall at shoulder height, fingers pointing upwards.
Your spine should be in a neutral position.

Movement: Begin by inhaling deeply.
As you exhale, bend your elbow and lean your torso towards the wall, as if you're trying to do a push-up against it. Ensure your elbow is pointing downwards and not flaring out to the sides.
Inhale as you push yourself back to the starting position, extending your arm fully.

Repeat with the other arm.

SCAN THE QR CODE
VIDEO EXPLANATION

ARMS/SHOULDER STRETCH

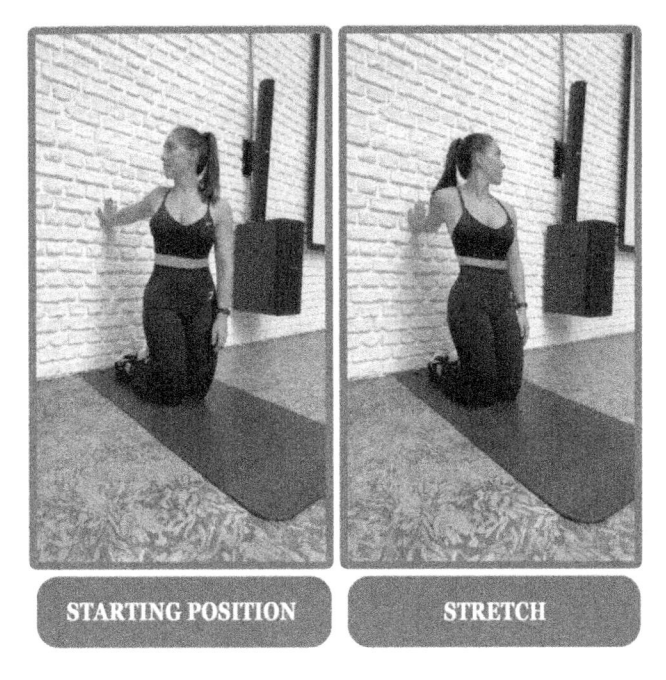

STARTING POSITION | **STRETCH**

Positioning: Stand sideways to the wall, about an arm's length away.

Initiation: Extend the arm closest to the wall straight out to the side at shoulder height and then place the palm flat against the wall. Your fingers should be pointing behind you.

Stretch: Gently turn your body away from the wall until you feel a stretch across the front of your shoulder and into the chest. Ensure that your arm remains flat against the wall and your body is upright, not leaning forward or backward.

Breathing: Take deep breaths, inhaling through the nose and exhaling through the mouth. With each exhale, try to deepen the stretch slightly, but without forcing or causing any pain.

SCAN THE QR CODE
VIDEO EXPLANATION

WALL PUSH-UPS

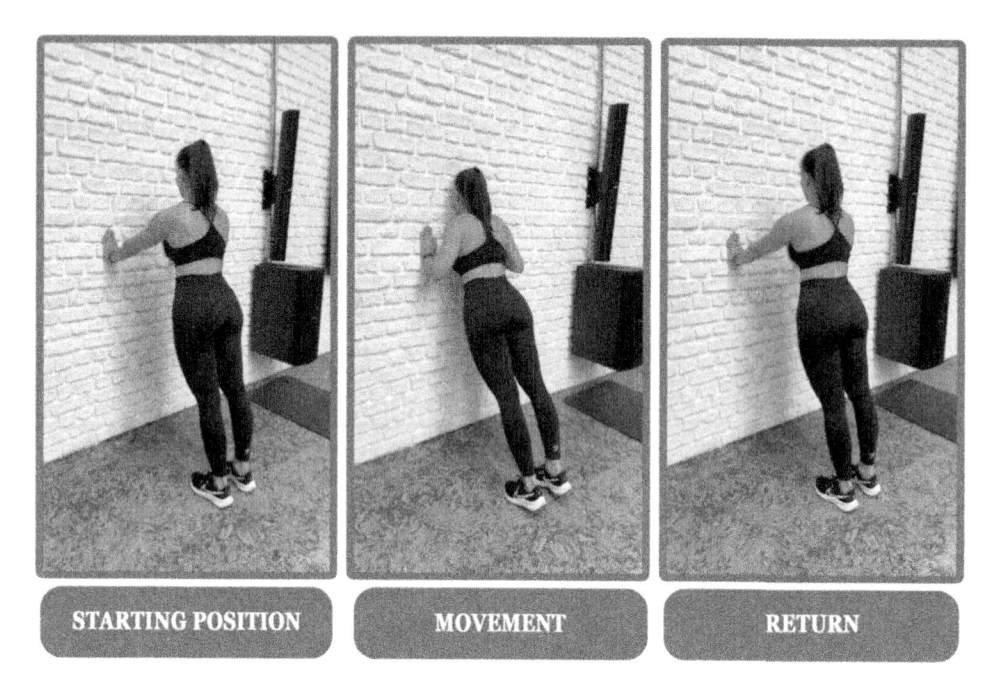

STARTING POSITION | **MOVEMENT** | **RETURN**

Positioning: Stand facing a wall, about an arm's length away. Place your hands on the wall slightly wider than shoulder-width apart and at chest height.

Movement: Keeping your body in a straight line from head to heels, bend your elbows and lean your body towards the wall. Ensure your elbows are angled slightly towards your body and not flaring out to the sides.

Engage the Core: As with all Pilates exercises, engage your core muscles to maintain stability and alignment. This not only strengthens the core but also protects the lower back.

Return: Push yourself back to the starting position by straightening your arms.

Breathing: Inhale as you bend your elbows and move towards the wall, and exhale as you push yourself back to the starting position.

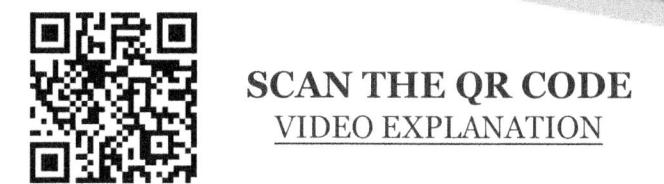

WALL PUSH-UPS DOG POSE VERSION

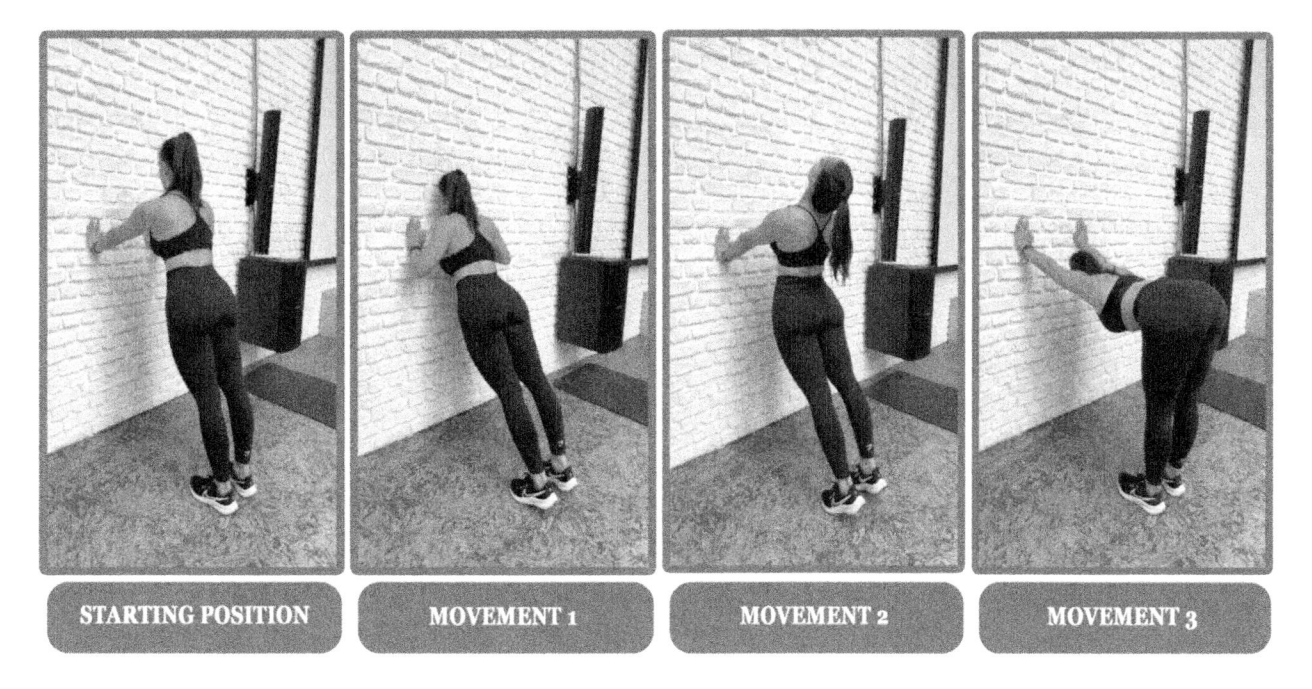

STARTING POSITION   **MOVEMENT 1**   **MOVEMENT 2**   **MOVEMENT 3**

Starting Position: Position yourself a short distance away from the wall, legs unified and arms outstretched as depicted.

Movement 1: Lean forward to touch your elbows to the wall, maintaining a straight back and legs.

Movement 2: Revert to your starting stance. Curve your back slightly by drawing your chest nearer to the wall and lifting your head, keeping your lower body stable. Pause in this posture briefly.

Movement 3: Finally, lean forward again, hands still in contact with the wall, and direct your gaze downward.

SCAN THE QR CODE
VIDEO EXPLANATION

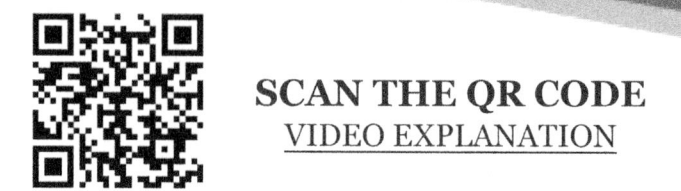

SEATED TRUNK ROTATION

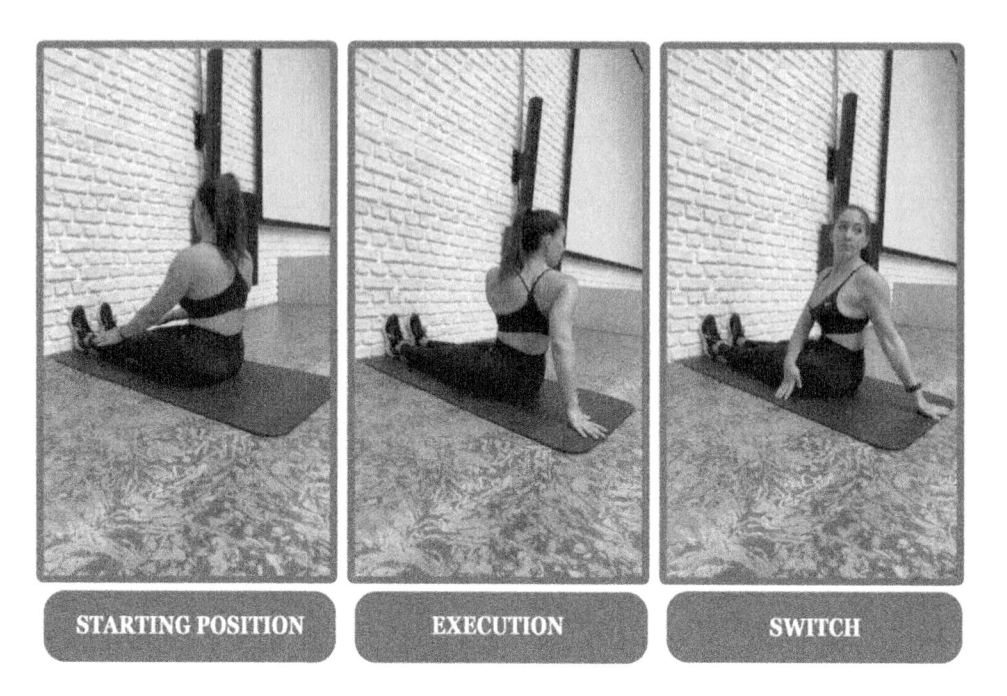

| STARTING POSITION | EXECUTION | SWITCH |

Starting Position: Begin by sitting on the floor with your legs extended straight in front of you. The soles of your feet should be touching the wall, and your heels should be pressed against it. Sit tall, ensuring your spine is elongated and your shoulders are relaxed.

Hand Placement: Place your hands behind you with your elbows pointing out to the sides. This position helps to keep the chest open and encourages rotation from the thoracic spine.

Movement: Inhale deeply. As you exhale, rotate your trunk to the right, aiming to bring your left elbow closer to your right knee. Ensure the rotation is coming from your waist and thoracic spine, not just your shoulders. Your feet should remain pressed against the wall, providing stability.

Hold and Return: Hold the rotated position for a moment, feeling the engagement of your obliques. Inhale as you slowly return to the center.

Repeat: Perform the same rotation to the left side, trying to bring your right elbow closer to your left knee.

SCAN THE QR CODE
VIDEO EXPLANATION

WALL TOUCHES PLANK

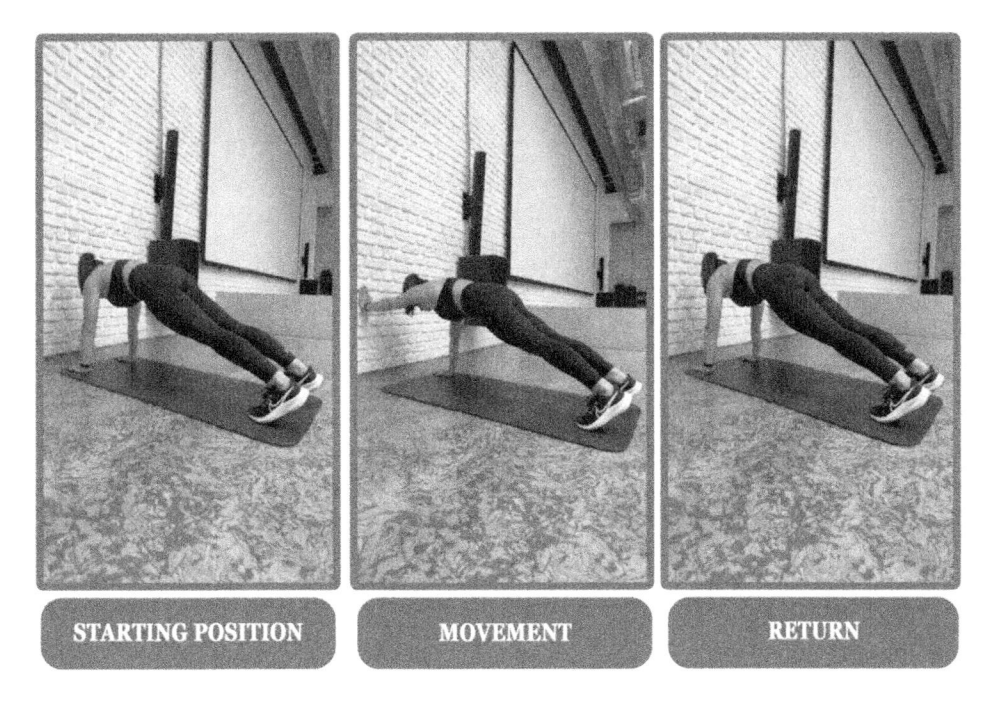

STARTING POSITION | **MOVEMENT** | **RETURN**

Starting Position: Begin in a traditional plank position, facing away from the wall. Your hands should be directly under your shoulders, and your body should form a straight line from your head to your heels.

Engage Core: Ensure your core is engaged, your back is flat, and your hips are level with the rest of your body.

Touch the Wall: While maintaining the plank position, lift one hand off the ground and touch the wall. The movement should be controlled, and the hips should remain as stable as possible to avoid rocking side to side.

Return to Starting Position: Bring the hand back to its starting position and repeat the movement with the opposite hand.

SCAN THE QR CODE
VIDEO EXPLANATION

EXTENDED DOWNWARD PLANK

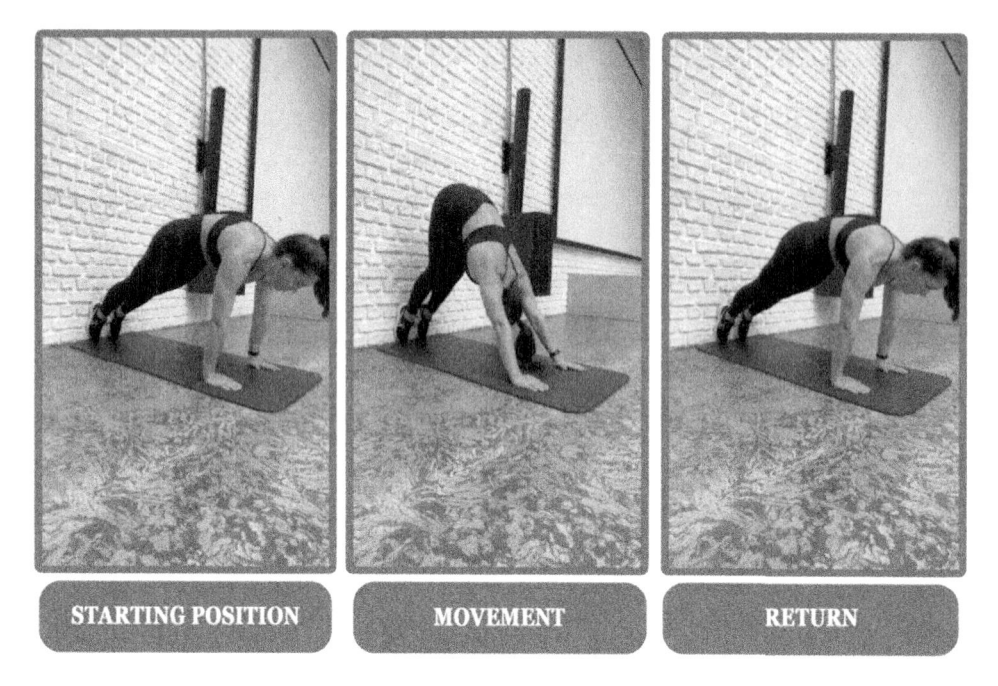

STARTING POSITION — **MOVEMENT** — **RETURN**

Plank Position: Begin by placing yourself in a plank position. Ensure your arms are straight and directly below your shoulders. The soles of your feet should be pressed firmly against the wall, and your body should form a straight line from your head to your heels.

Transition to Downward Dog: From the plank position, slowly and controlled, raise your hips towards the ceiling, forming a V-shape with your body. This is similar to the Downward Dog position in yoga. As you do this, ensure your arms and legs remain straight. A minimal bend at the knees is acceptable if needed for comfort or flexibility reasons.

Hold and Return: Hold the V-shaped position for a second, ensuring you maintain steady breathing. After the brief pause, gradually lower your hips and return to the initial plank position.

LOWER BODY EXERCISES

SCAN THE QR CODE
VIDEO EXPLANATION

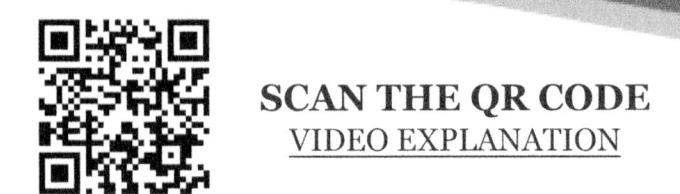

WALL HIP THRUST / BRIDGE WITH BOTH LEGS

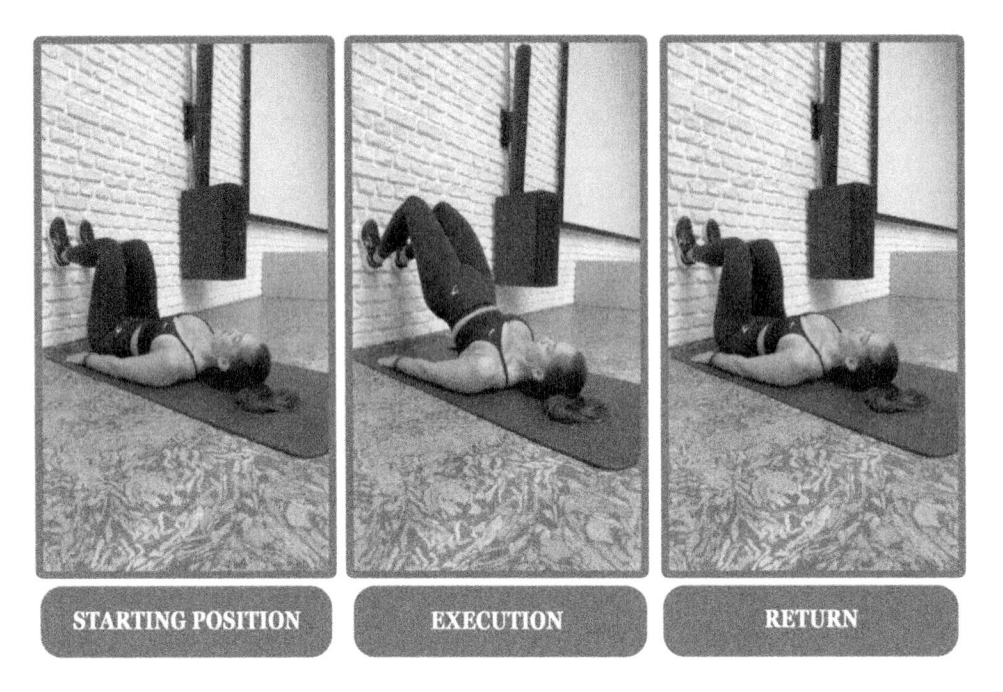

| STARTING POSITION | EXECUTION | RETURN |

Starting Position: Begin by lying flat on your back on the ground, with your feet propped against the wall and knees forming a 90-degree angle. Place your arms beside you.

Execution: From this initial stance, elevate your hips while engaging your glute muscles.

Return: Return to your starting position and continue to perform the movement for the specified number of repetitions in your exercise plan.

SCAN THE QR CODE
VIDEO EXPLANATION

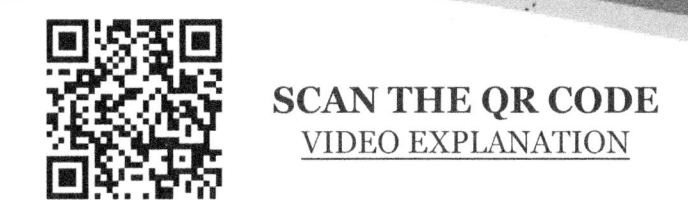

LUNGES CLASSIC

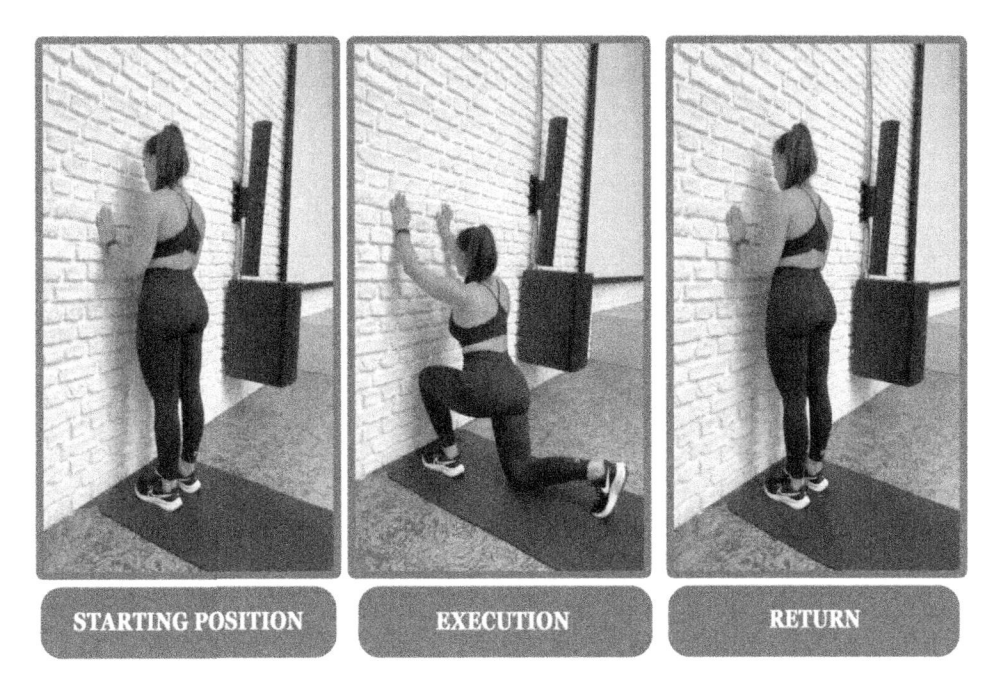

STARTING POSITION | **EXECUTION** | **RETURN**

Starting Position: Stand facing a wall

Execution: Extend your right leg back. Lightly use your fingertips for wall support. Maintain a straight posture for both your back and arms. Lower yourself into the lunge, bringing your right knee close to the ground. Hold this stance briefly while keeping your back and arms aligned.

Return: Return to your starting position and continue to perform the movement for the specified number of repetitions in your exercise plan.

Do the same with the other leg.

SCAN THE QR CODE
VIDEO EXPLANATION

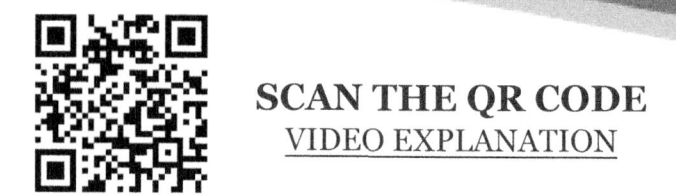

LUNGES + KICK BACK

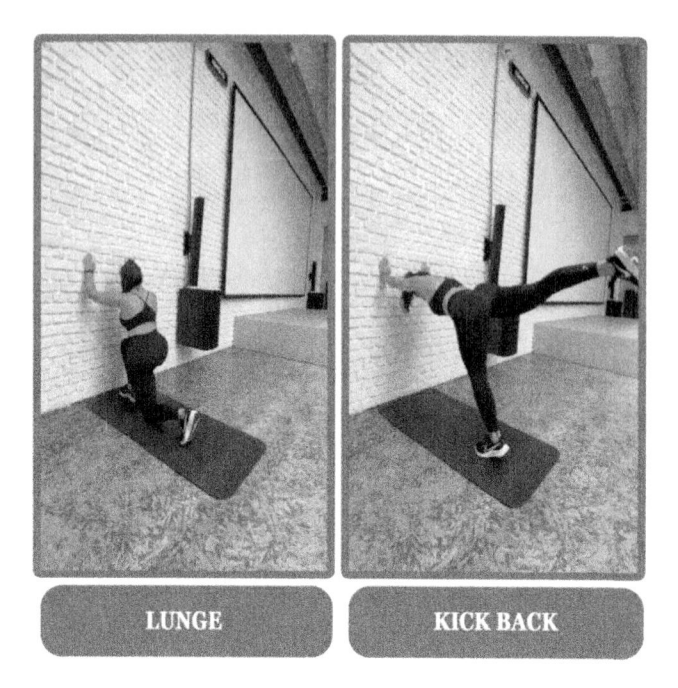

LUNGE | **KICK BACK**

Starting Position: To perform wall-assisted lunges, position yourself facing the wall.

Lunge: Extend your right leg forward and your left leg back. Use both hands to grip the wall securely. Keep your spine aligned.

Kick Back: Gradually rise onto your tiptoes and then extend your right leg backward. Ensure your back, head, shoulders, hips, and legs form a straight line. Keep your arms extended and your hands anchored to the wall. Hold this stance briefly before reverting to your starting position.

Do the same with the other leg

SCAN THE QR CODE
VIDEO EXPLANATION

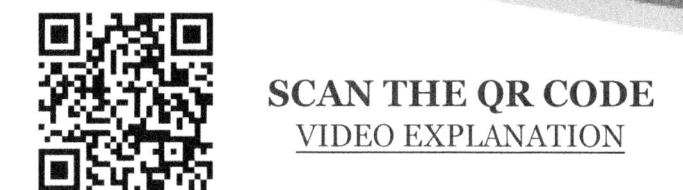

BACK TO THE WALL LUNGES

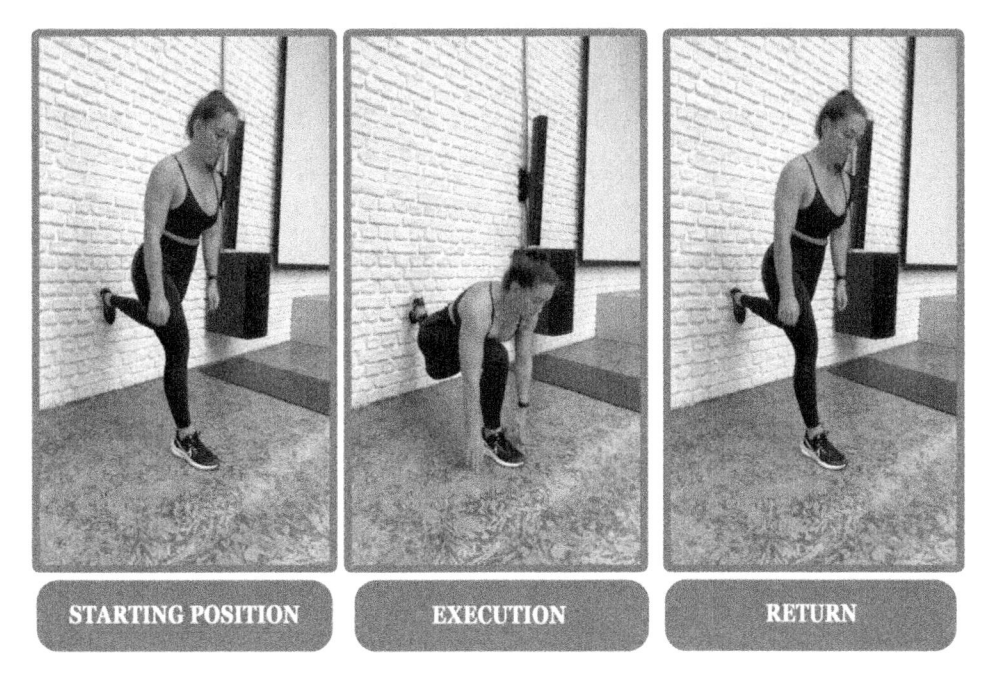

STARTING POSITION | **EXECUTION** | **RETURN**

Starting Position: Extend your right knee forward while your left toes touch the wall, knee bent.

Execution: Keep your arms hanging down and your back upright.

Return: Gradually rise, lifting your left knee off the wall but keeping your toes in contact.

Do the same with the other leg

SCAN THE QR CODE
VIDEO EXPLANATION

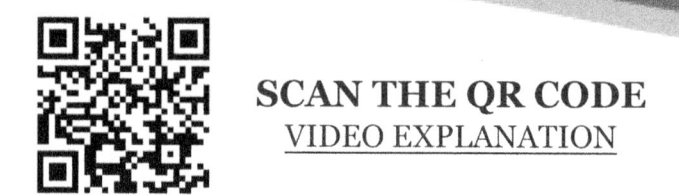

WALL SQUATS

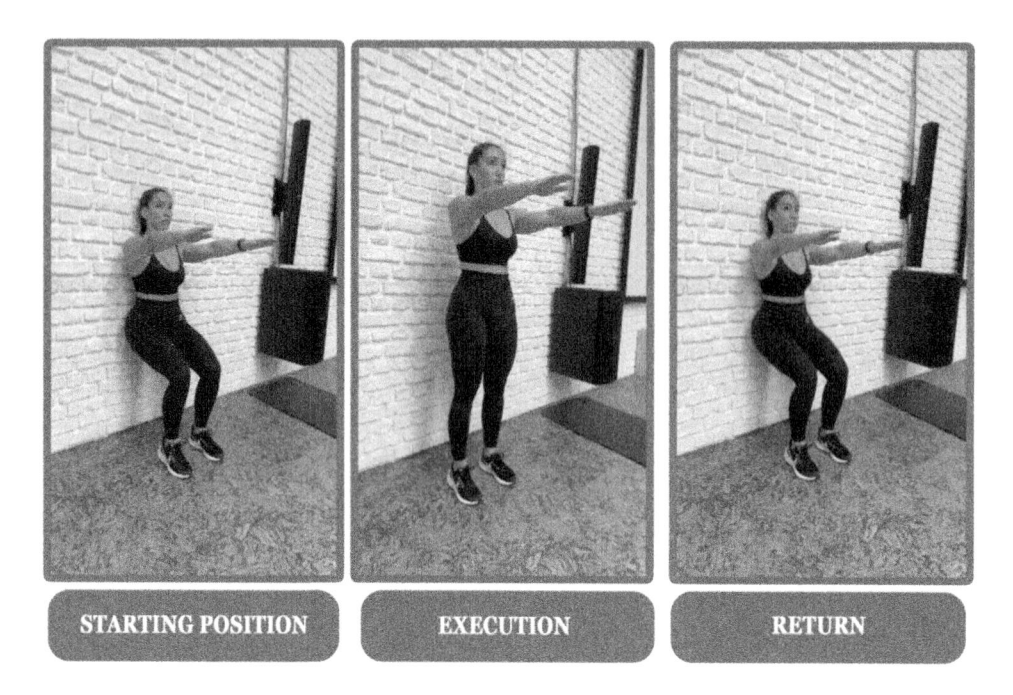

STARTING POSITION | **EXECUTION** | **RETURN**

* In this exercise, there can be 2 variations. One where you do the squat sliding against the wall and one where you detach from the wall to perform the squat. In the illustration and in the video, I'm showing variation number 2.
Now I'll explain variation number 1. Choose the one you prefer:

Positioning: Stand with your back against a wall, feet hip-width apart and positioned about 2 feet away from the wall. Your arms can be by your sides or extended out in front of you for balance.

Execution: Slide your back down the wall, bending your knees and lowering your body into a squat position. Your knees should be directly above your ankles, forming a 90-degree angle. Ensure that your back remains flat against the wall throughout the movement.

Hold & Return: Maintain the squat position for a set duration, engaging your core and keeping your thighs parallel to the ground. The challenge is to hold the position while maintaining proper form. Slowly slide back up the wall to return to the starting position.

SCAN THE QR CODE
VIDEO EXPLANATION

WALL SIT HEEL RAISE

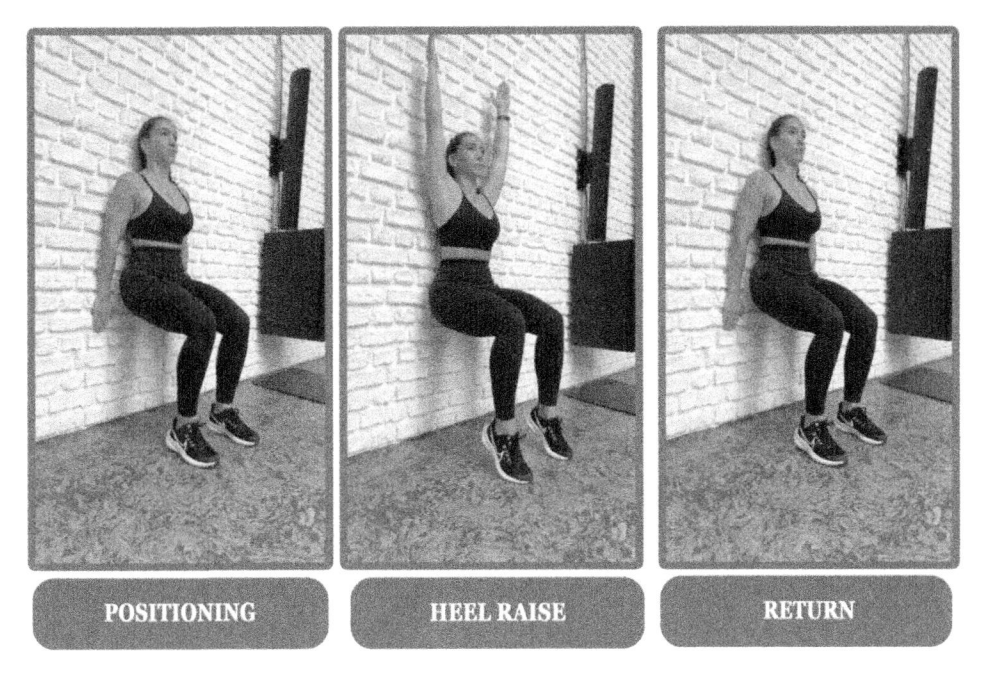

| POSITIONING | HEEL RAISE | RETURN |

Positioning: Stand with your back against a wall. Walk your feet out in front of you and slide your back down the wall until your thighs are parallel to the ground, as if you're sitting in an invisible chair. Your knees should be directly above your ankles, forming a 90-degree angle. Press your lower back into the wall for support.

Heel Raise: While maintaining the wall sit position, slowly lift both heels off the ground, rising onto the balls of your feet. This will engage your calf muscles.

Return: Slowly lower your heels back to the ground.

SCAN THE QR CODE
VIDEO EXPLANATION

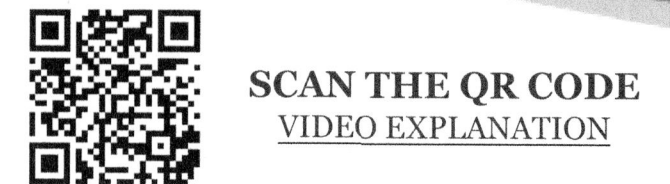

STANDING WALL LEG LIFT

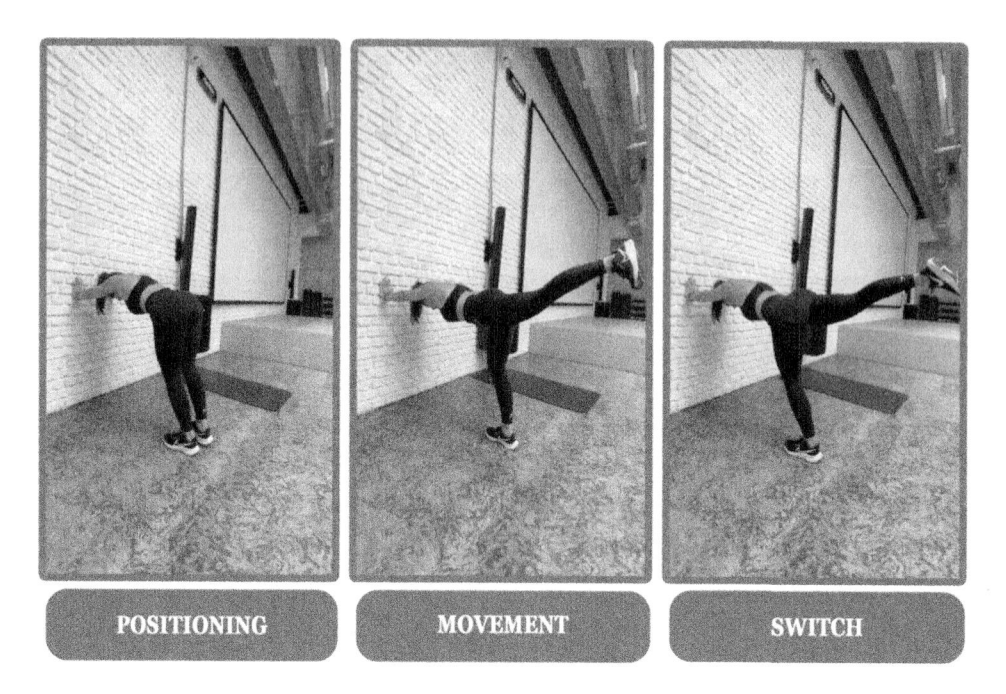

POSITIONING | MOVEMENT | SWITCH

Positioning: Stand facing away from the wall, about a foot or two away, depending on your height and flexibility. Place both hands on the wall, either directly beneath your shoulders or slightly in front of you, depending on your comfort. Your body should be in a slight diagonal line from head to heels.

Movement: Engage your core and keep your back straight. Lift one leg and extend it straight back, trying to bring it parallel to the ground or as high as your flexibility allows. The sole of your foot should be facing the ceiling, and your toes pointed. Ensure your hips remain square to the ground, avoiding any rotation.

Return and Repeat: Slowly lower the leg back down and repeat the movement with the other leg.

SCAN THE QR CODE
VIDEO EXPLANATION

CLAMSHELLS

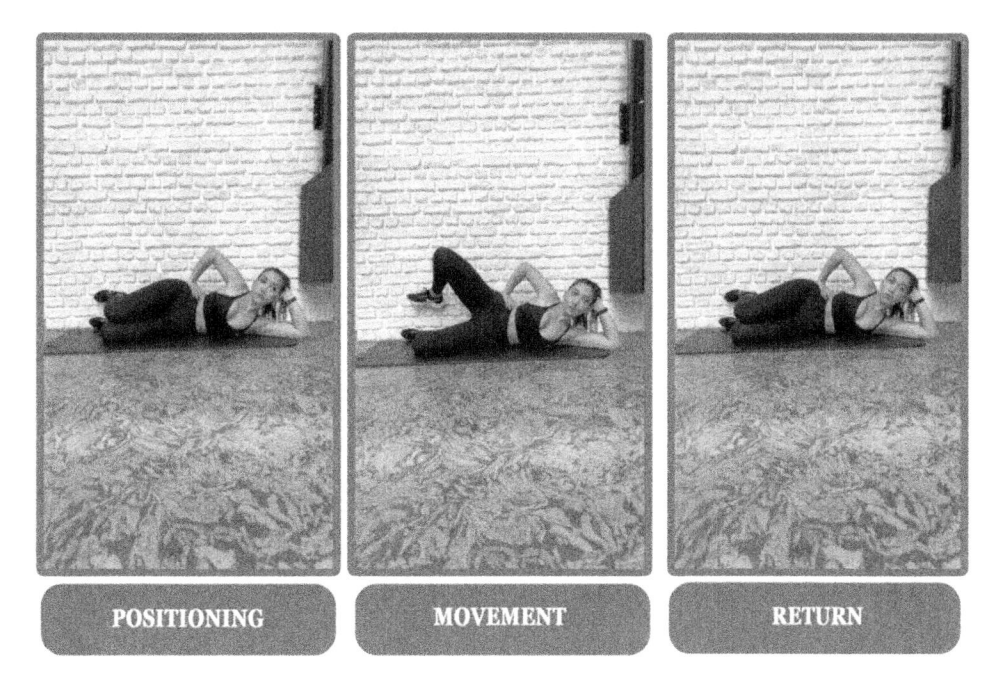

| POSITIONING | MOVEMENT | RETURN |

Positioning: Begin by lying on your side with your back against the wall. Your hips and knees should be bent at a 90-degree angle, and your feet should be stacked and in line with your glutes, resting against the wall.

Engage Core: Before initiating the movement, engage your core muscles to stabilize your spine and pelvis.

Movement: Keeping your feet together and pressed against the wall, lift your top knee as high as you can without moving your pelvis or lower back. Your legs will resemble a clam opening, hence the name. The wall provides resistance as you lift your knee, making the exercise more challenging.

Return: Slowly lower your knee back down, ensuring that you maintain control throughout the movement.

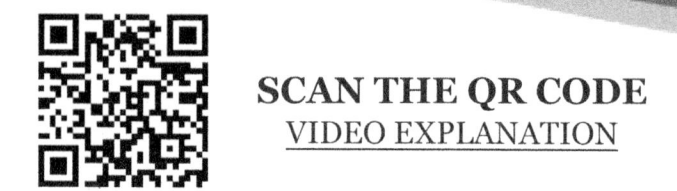

FORWARD WALL SQUATS

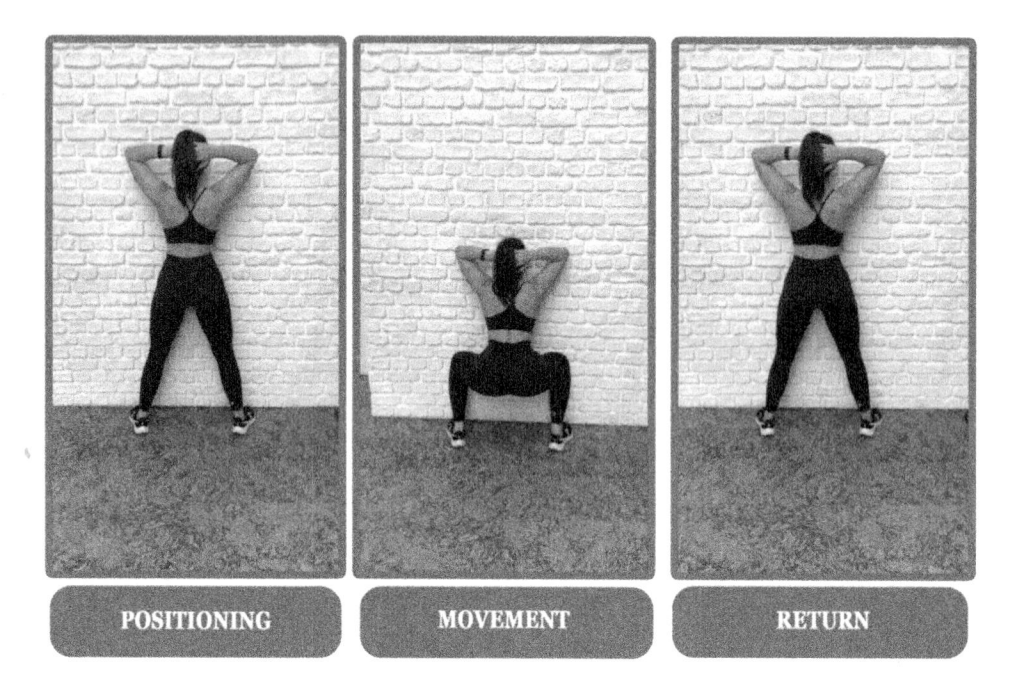

POSITIONING — MOVEMENT — RETURN

Positioning: Stand facing the wall, with your toes and nose almost touching it. Your feet should be hip-width apart or slightly wider. (see illustration)

Starting Position: Keep your arms behind your head. Your posture should be upright with your chest lifted.

Movement: Begin to lower your body into a squat position, bending your knees and pushing your hips back as if you're sitting in a chair. As you descend, ensure that your knees don't move past your toes. Given the close proximity to the wall, it's crucial to maintain an upright posture to avoid leaning into the wall.

Return: Press through your heels to stand back up, straightening your legs and returning to the starting position.

SCAN THE QR CODE
VIDEO EXPLANATION

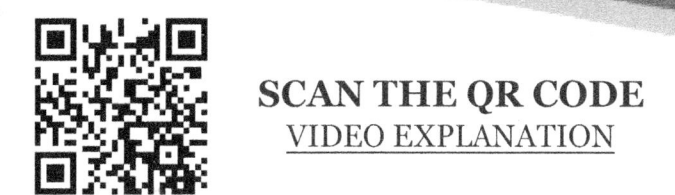

ONE-LEGGED WALL SIT

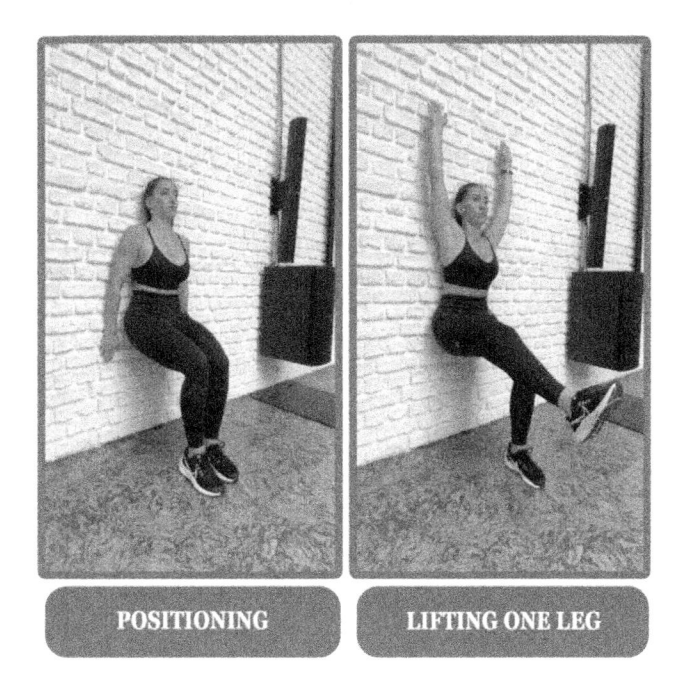

Positioning: Start by standing with your back against a wall. Your feet should be about hip-width apart and positioned approximately 2 feet away from the wall.
Slide your back down the wall, bending your knees until they are at a 90-degree angle, as if you're sitting in an invisible chair. Your thighs should be parallel to the ground, and your knees should be directly above your ankles.

Lifting One Leg: Once you're in the wall sit position, slowly lift one foot off the ground, extending it straight out in front of you. Keep the foot flexed and try to maintain a straight line from your hip to your heel.

Holding: Engage your core and press your back firmly against the wall. Hold this position for a set duration or as long as you can maintain good form.

Switching: Return the lifted leg to the ground and repeat the exercise with the other leg.

SCAN THE QR CODE
VIDEO EXPLANATION

GLUTE BRIDGE HALF-ASSISTED

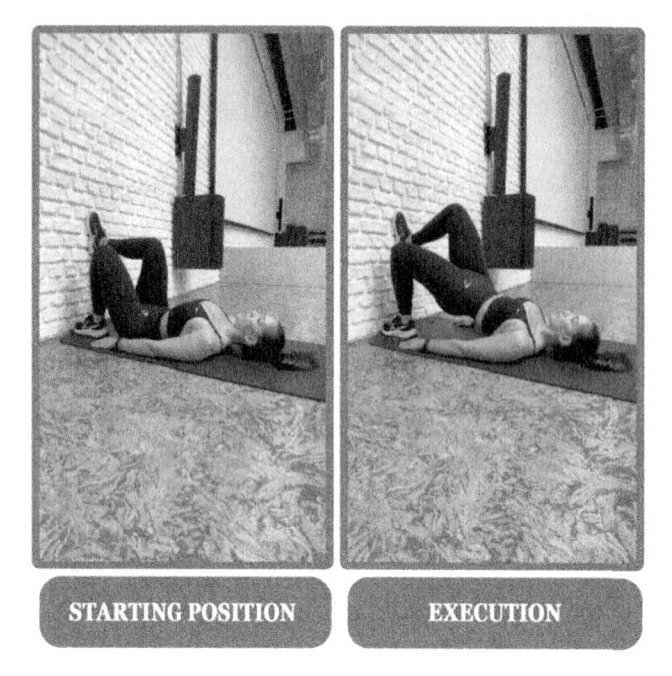

STARTING POSITION **EXECUTION**

Starting Position: Lie on your back on a mat or comfortable surface, facing away from the wall. Place one foot flat on the wall with the knee bent, while the other foot remains flat on the floor, also with the knee bent. Ensure both feet are hip-width apart.
Arms should be at your sides, palms facing down.

Execution: Engage your core and press your palms into the floor for stability.
Push through the heel on the wall and the foot on the floor simultaneously, lifting your hips off the ground. As you do this, squeeze your glutes and ensure your body forms a straight line from your shoulders to your knees.
Hold the bridge position for a moment, ensuring your hips are lifted and glutes are engaged.
Slowly lower your hips back to the starting position. Switch to the other leg.

SCAN THE QR CODE
VIDEO EXPLANATION

SINGLE LEG GLUTE BRIDGE

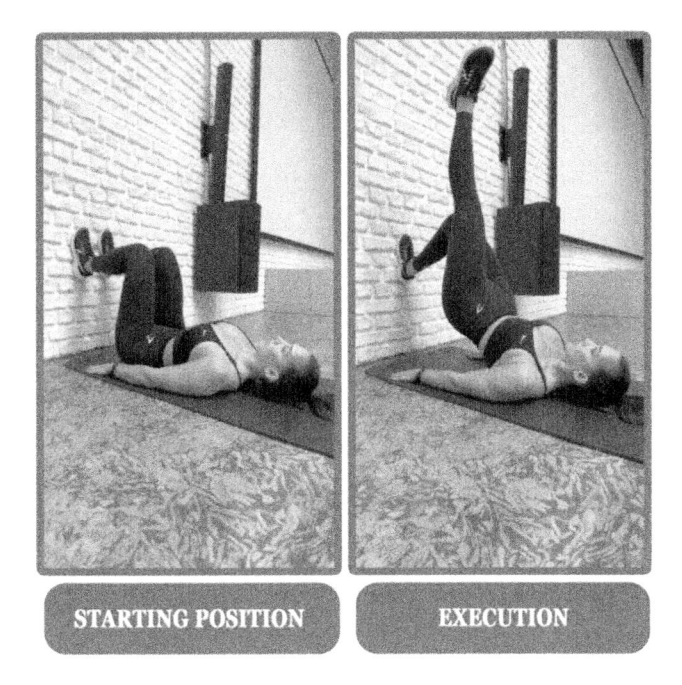

STARTING POSITION | **EXECUTION**

Starting Position: Lie on your back on a mat, with your arms at your sides. Place the heel of one foot firmly against the wall, with the knee bent at approximately a 90-degree angle. Extend the other leg straight up towards the ceiling.

Movement: Pressing through the heel that's on the wall, lift your hips off the ground by squeezing your glutes. The aim is to create a straight line from the shoulders to the knee of the bent leg. The extended leg will move upward as your hips rise.

Hold and Lower: At the top of the movement, ensure your hips are level and you're not arching your back. Hold the position for a moment, feeling the contraction in your glutes and hamstrings. Slowly lower your hips back down to the starting position. Switch to the other leg.

FLEXIBILITY AND BALANCE EXERCISES

SCAN THE QR CODE
VIDEO EXPLANATION

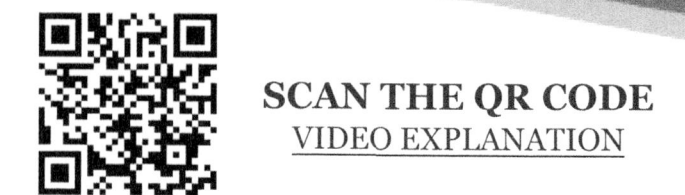

WALL SIDE LEG LIFT

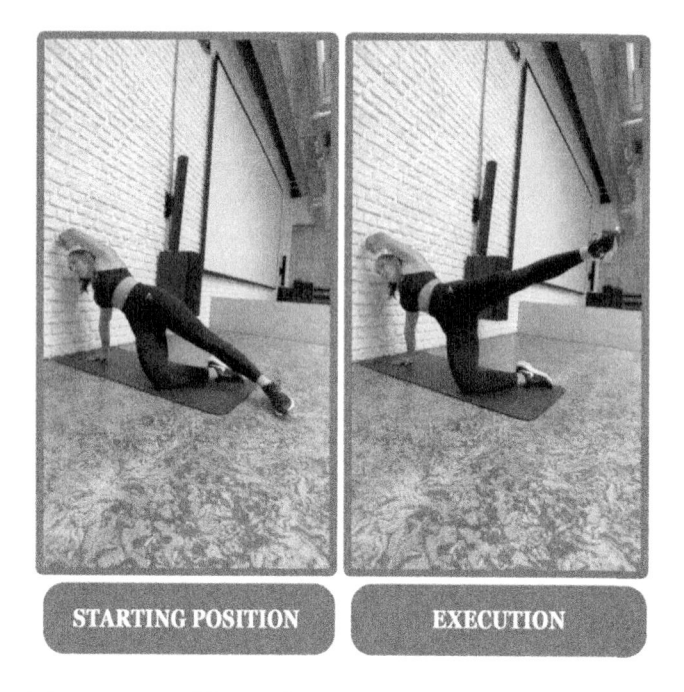

STARTING POSITION **EXECUTION**

Starting Position: Position yourself on the mat so that your right knee and right hand are touching it.

Execution: Place your left hand firmly against the wall and stretch your left leg out so it's level with the ground. Begin lifting and lowering your leg without letting it touch the floor. Perform the same movements with your opposite leg.

SCAN THE QR CODE
VIDEO EXPLANATION

TOE TOUCH CRUNCH

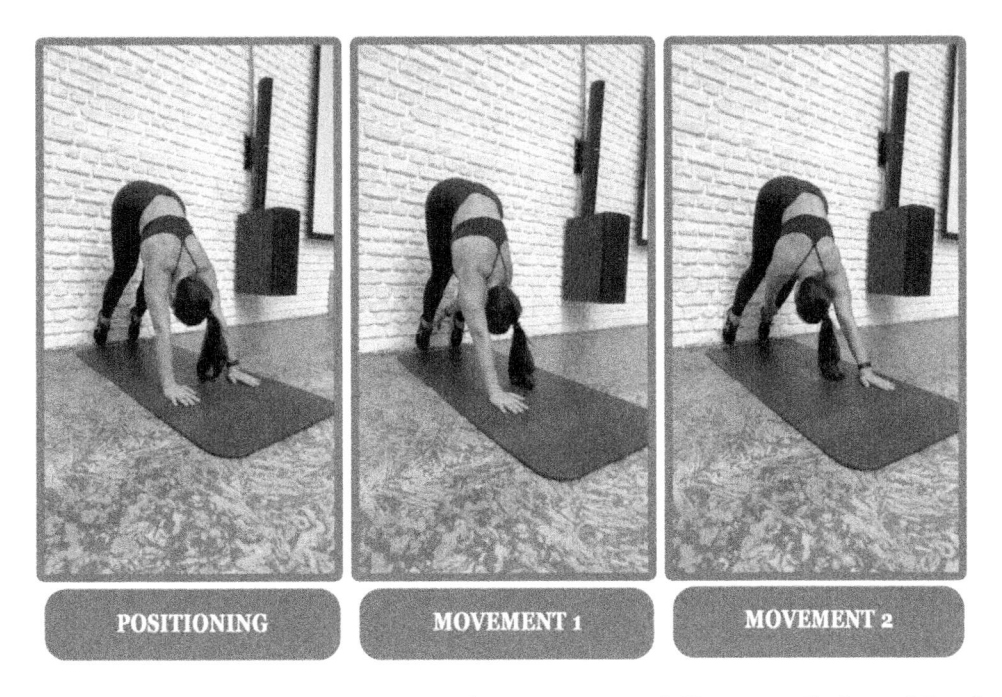

| POSITIONING | MOVEMENT 1 | MOVEMENT 2 |

Starting Position: Stand facing away from the mat, arms fully extended, and heels touching the wall.

Movement 1: On an exhale, elevate your hips and reach your left hand to your right ankle.
Inhale as you revert to the initial pose.

Movement 2: Exhale again, this time lifting your hips and connecting your right hand to your left ankle.
Inhale to return to your starting stance.

SCAN THE QR CODE
VIDEO EXPLANATION

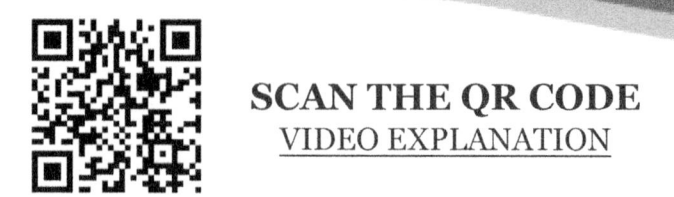

WALL TABLE TOP

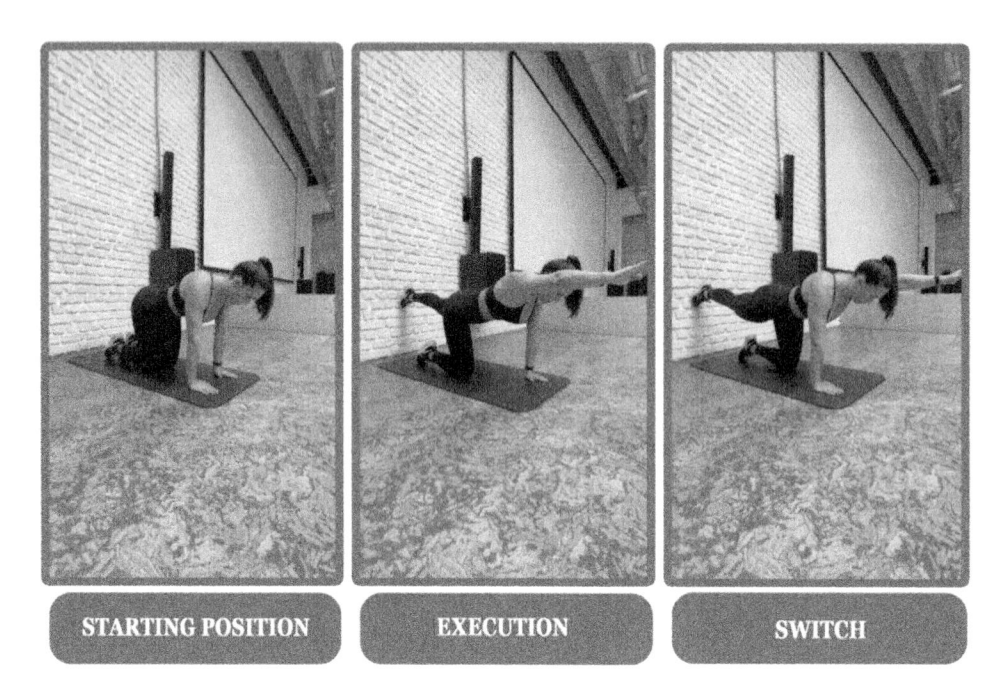

| STARTING POSITION | EXECUTION | SWITCH |

Starting Position: Start in a kneeling position, with your arms extended and hands resting on the ground. As with all Pilates exercises, begin by taking a deep breath and engaging your core muscles, ensuring your spine remains in a neutral position throughout the movement.

Execution: Leg Elevation - Slowly lift one leg, trying to touch the wall with your foot. The height of the elevation will depend on your flexibility and strength. Ideally, you want your shin to be parallel to the ground or as close to it as you can get.
Opposite Arm Elevation - As you lift your leg to touch the wall, simultaneously raise the opposite arm until it's parallel to the ground. Your palm should face down, and your arm should be straight.

Hold and Breathe: In this position, with one leg elevated and touching the wall and the opposite arm raised and parallel to the ground, hold for a few breaths. Ensure your core remains engaged and your balance is steady. Slowly lower your leg and arm back to the starting position.

Repeat: Perform the same movement on the opposite side, lifting the other leg and the opposite arm.

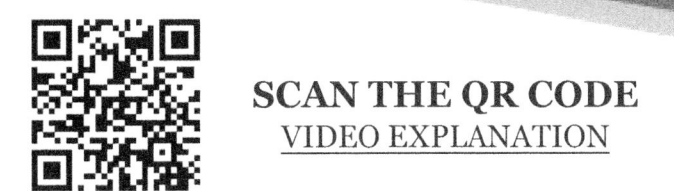

WALL SINGLE LEG STRETCH (LEFT & RIGHT)

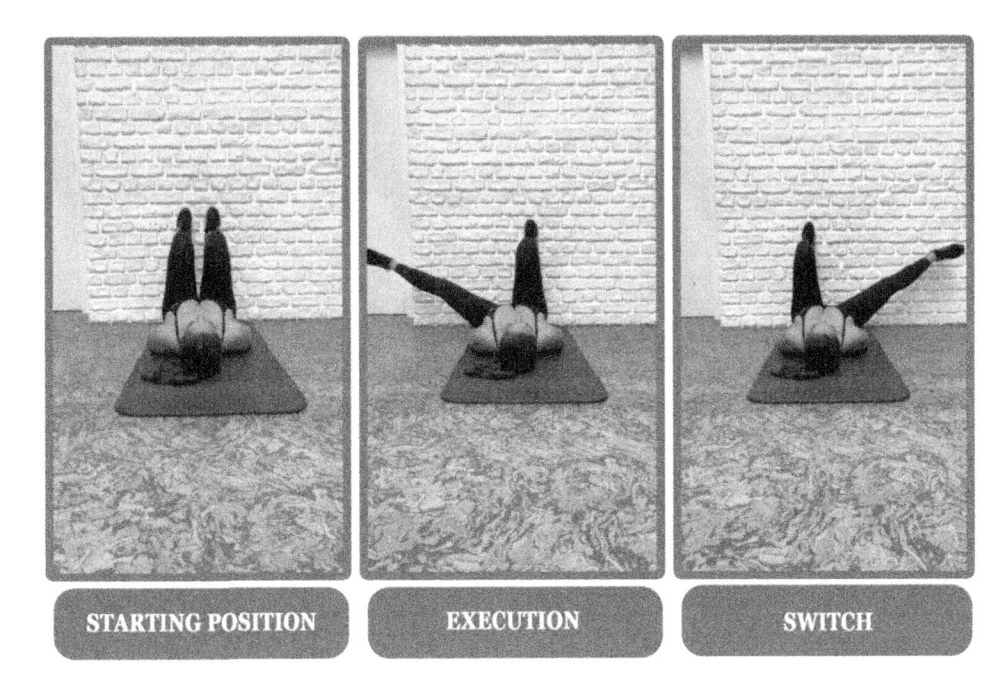

STARTING POSITION   **EXECUTION**   **SWITCH**

Starting Position: Start by lying flat on the ground with your feet against the wall, knees bent at roughly a 90-degree angle.

Execution: Extend your left leg skyward. Initiate a lateral movement to the left while keeping your leg straight and muscles engaged. Aim to feel a stretch along the inner part of your left thigh. Extend your leg as far to the side as your flexibility allows. Coordinate your breathing by inhaling when lifting your leg and exhaling as you move it sideways.

WALL SCISSOR

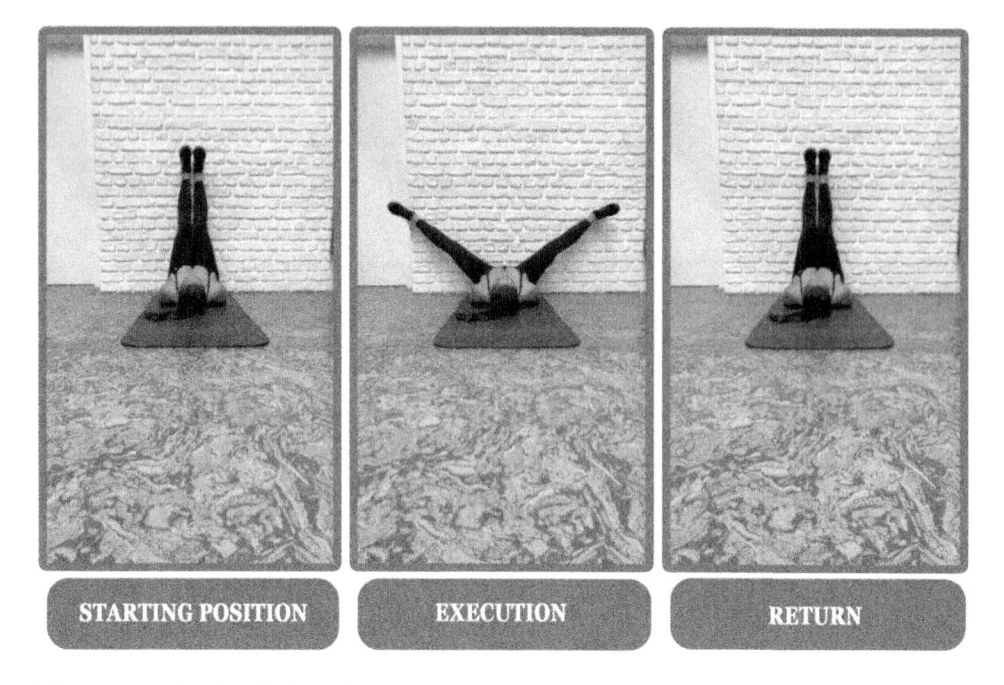

STARTING POSITION | **EXECUTION** | **RETURN**

Starting Position: Begin by lying flat on a mat, ensuring your lower back is flush against the wall. Elevate your legs and keep them close together.

Execution: Then, separate your legs to the maximum extent, pulling your feet apart. Maintain this stance for a 5-second count.

Return: Finally, bring your legs back together and ease your muscles, returning to the initial position.

SCAN THE QR CODE
<u>VIDEO EXPLANATION</u>

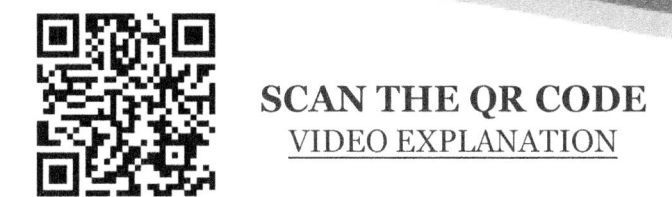

EXTENDED GLUTE BRIDGE ROTATION

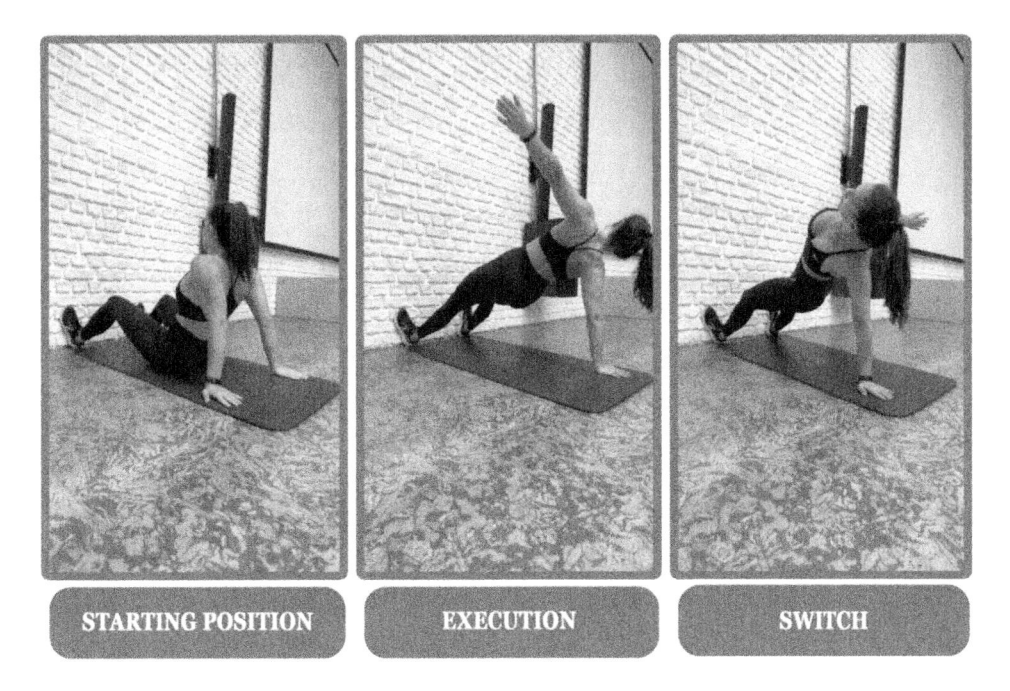

STARTING POSITION | **EXECUTION** | **SWITCH**

Starting Position: Begin by sitting near a wall with your feet touching the wall. Position your left hand slightly to the side behind you, maintaining an upright torso and elevated chest.

Execution: Keeping your limbs straight, elevate your hips off the ground as high as possible while simultaneously reaching your left arm towards the ceiling.

Maintain this pose for a one-second count, then revert to your initial position. Complete the designated number of repetitions on one side before switching to the other.

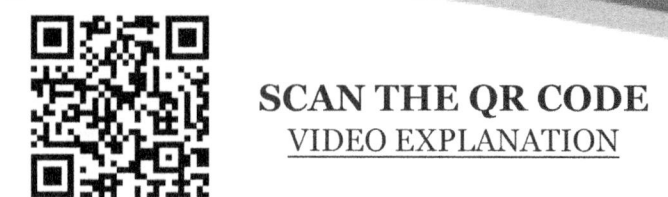

DYNAMIC PLANK WITH WALL SUPPORT

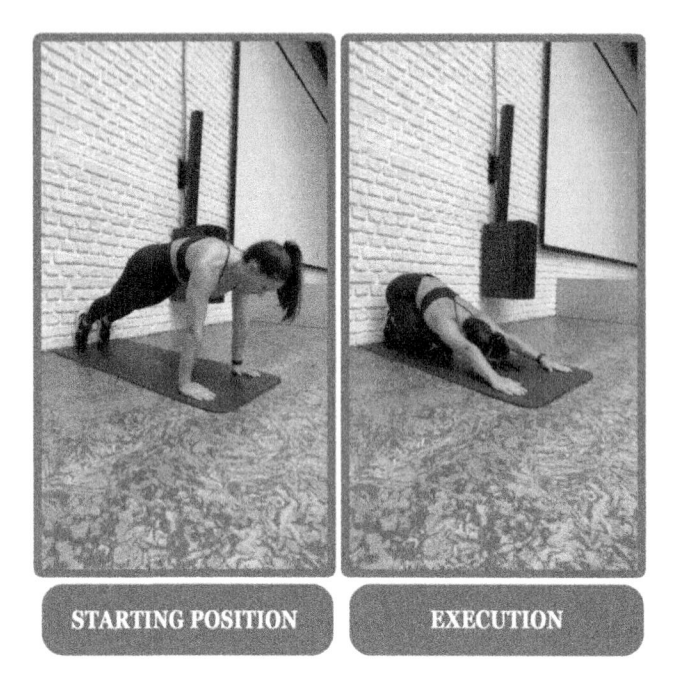

STARTING POSITION | **EXECUTION**

Starting Position: Begin by getting into a plank stance, positioning your feet against the wall. Your toes should touch the ground while the soles are against the wall. Maintain a straight body line and align your hands directly under your shoulders.

Execution: Next, draw your hips back towards the wall by bending your knees. As you do this, keep your arms extended and experience a stretch along your back. Hold this position for a brief second.

Return: Finally, revert to your initial plank position. Continue to perform the exercise for the specified number of repetitions or duration.

Chapter 5: Specialized Workout Programs

IMPORTANT: If after finishing your workout you don't feel particularly tired, you can move on to the intermediate one or repeat the daily workout up to a maximum of 3 times.

WARM UP ROUTINE (10 MINS)

What I recommend is to include these exercises every time you start a workout. Then conclude it with some Cooldown exercises.

MONDAY:

Wall Mountain Climbers - 1 minute | **PAGE 20**

Wall lateral Lunges - 1 minute (30 seconds each side) | **PAGE 21**

Wall Leg Swings - 1 minute (30 seconds front/back, 30 seconds side-to-side) | **PAGE 22**

Wall Single-Leg Lifts - 1 minute (30 seconds each leg) | **PAGE 23**

Arm Circles - 1 minute (30 seconds forward, 30 seconds backward) | **PAGE 25**

Repeat the routine once more.

TUESDAY:

Wall Angels - 1 minute | **PAGE 27**

Knee to Nose - 1 minute | **PAGE 28**

Wall Leg Raise + Kick Back - 1 minute (30 seconds each leg) | **PAGE 29**

Wall Single Leg Circles - 1 minute (30 seconds each leg) | **PAGE 26**

Wall Calf Raises - 1 minute | **PAGE 24**

Repeat the routine once more.

WEDNESDAY:

Wall lateral Lunges - 1 minute (30 seconds each side) | **PAGE 21**

Wall Mountain Climbers - 1 minute | **PAGE 20**

Wall Leg Swings - 1 minute (30 seconds front/back, 30 seconds side-to-side) | **PAGE 22**

Wall Single-Leg Lifts - 1 minute (30 seconds each leg) | **PAGE 23**

Wall Angels - 1 minute | **PAGE 27**

Repeat the routine once more.

THURSDAY:

Arm Circles - 1 minute (30 seconds forward, 30 seconds backward) | **PAGE 25**

Wall Single Leg Circles - 1 minute (30 seconds each leg) | **PAGE 26**

Wall Calf Raises - 1 minute | **PAGE 24**

Knee to Nose - 1 minute | **PAGE 28**

Wall Leg Raise + Kick Back - 1 minute (30 seconds each leg) | **PAGE 29**

Repeat the routine once more.

FRIDAY:

Wall Angels - 1 minute | **PAGE 27**

Wall Mountain Climbers - 1 minute | **PAGE 20**

Wall lateral Lunges - 1 minute (30 seconds each side) | **PAGE 21**

Wall Leg Swings - 1 minute (30 seconds front/back, 30 seconds side-to-side) | **PAGE 22**

Arm Circles - 1 minute (30 seconds forward, 30 seconds backward) | **PAGE 25**

Repeat the routine once more.

SATURDAY:

Wall Single-Leg Lifts - 1 minute (30 seconds each leg) | **PAGE 23**

Wall Calf Raises - 1 minute | **PAGE 24**

Wall Single Leg Circles - 1 minute (30 seconds each leg) | **PAGE 26**

Knee to Nose - 1 minute | **PAGE 28**

Wall Leg Raise + Kick Back - 1 minute (30 seconds each leg) | **PAGE 29**

Repeat the routine once more.

COOLDOWN ROUTINE

Wall Cobra Pose - 30 seconds: Stretches the chest, shoulders, and abs. | **PAGE 33**

Wall Cat Pose - 30 seconds: Mobilizes the spine. | **PAGE 34**

Wall-Assisted Puppy Pose – 30 seconds: Stretches the shoulders and spine. | **PAGE 36**

Lower Body Stretch – 30 seconds each: Targets the hamstrings, calves, and quadriceps. | **PAGE 35**

Wall Sphinx Pose – hold 30 seconds :Targets the erector spinae, trapezius, and rhomboids in the back, as well as the deltoids in the shoulders, you would also likely experience a stretch in the glutes and hamstrings. | **PAGE 37**

FLEXIBILITY FOCUS WEEKLY WORKOUT PLAN

BEGINNER LEVEL: FLEXIBILITY FOCUS

MONDAY:

Wall Mountain Climbers - 30 seconds | **PAGE 20**

Wall Leg Swings - 10 repetitions each leg | **PAGE 21**

Arm Circles - 30 seconds | **PAGE 25**

Wall Angels - 10 repetitions | **PAGE 27**

Arms/Shoulder Stretch - 30 seconds hold | **PAGE 53**

TUESDAY:

Wall lateral Lunges - 10 repetitions each side | **PAGE 21**

Wall Single-Leg Lifts - 10 repetitions each leg | **PAGE 22**

Knee to Nose - 10 repetitions | **PAGE 28**

Wall Side Leg Lift - 30 seconds each side | **PAGE 74**

Toe Touch Crunch - 10 repetitions | **PAGE 75**

WEDNESDAY:

Wall Calf Raises - 15 repetitions | **PAGE 24**

Wall Single Leg Circles - 10 repetitions each leg | **PAGE 26**

Wall Table Top - 30 seconds | **PAGE 76**

Wall Leg Raise + Kick Back - 10 repetitions | **PAGE 29**

Wall Scissor - 30 seconds | **PAGE 78**

THURSDAY:

Wall Mountain Climbers - 30 seconds | **PAGE 20**

Wall Leg Swings - 10 repetitions each leg | **PAGE 22**

Arm Circles - 30 seconds | **PAGE 25**

Wall Angels - 10 repetitions | **PAGE 27**

Arms/Shoulder Stretch - 30 seconds hold | **PAGE 53**

FRIDAY:

Wall lateral Lunges - 10 repetitions each side | **PAGE 21**

Wall Single-Leg Lifts - 10 repetitions each leg | **PAGE 23**

Knee to Nose - 10 repetitions | **PAGE 28**

Wall Side Leg Lift - 30 seconds each side | **PAGE 74**

Toe Touch Crunch - 10 repetitions | **PAGE 75**

SATURDAY:

Wall Calf Raises - 15 repetitions | **PAGE 24**

Wall Single Leg Circles - 10 repetitions each leg | **PAGE 26**

Wall Table Top - 30 seconds | **PAGE 76**

Wall Leg Raise + Kick Back - 10 repetitions | **PAGE 29**

Wall Scissor - 30 seconds | **PAGE 78**

INTERMEDIATE LEVEL: FLEXIBILITY FOCUS

MONDAY:

Wall Mountain Climbers - 45 seconds | **PAGE 20**

Wall Leg Swings - 15 repetitions each leg | **PAGE 22**

Arm Circles - 45 seconds | **PAGE 25**

Wall Angels - 15 repetitions | **PAGE 27**

Extended Glute Bridge Rotation - 30 seconds | **PAGE 79**

TUESDAY:

Wall lateral Lunges - 15 repetitions each side | **PAGE 21**

Wall Single-Leg Lifts - 15 repetitions each leg | **PAGE 23**

Knee to Nose - 15 repetitions | **PAGE 28**

Wall Side Leg Lift - 45 seconds each side | **PAGE 74**

Dynamic Plank with Wall Support - 30 seconds | **PAGE 80**

WEDNESDAY:

Wall Calf Raises - 20 repetitions | **PAGE 24**

Wall Single Leg Circles - 15 repetitions each leg | **PAGE 26**

Wall Table Top - 45 seconds | **PAGE 76**

Wall Leg Raise + Kick Back - 15 repetitions | **PAGE 29**

Wall Scissor - 45 seconds | **PAGE 78**

THURSDAY:

Wall Mountain Climbers - 45 seconds | **PAGE 20**

Wall Leg Swings - 15 repetitions each leg | **PAGE 22**

Arm Circles - 45 seconds | **PAGE 25**

Wall Angels - 15 repetitions | **PAGE 27**

Extended Glute Bridge Rotation - 30 seconds | **PAGE 79**

FRIDAY:

Wall lateral Lunges - 15 repetitions each side | **PAGE 21**

Wall Single-Leg Lifts - 15 repetitions each leg | **PAGE 23**

Knee to Nose - 15 repetitions | **PAGE 28**

Wall Side Leg Lift - 45 seconds each side | **PAGE 74**

Dynamic Plank with Wall Support - 30 seconds | **PAGE 80**

SATURDAY:

Wall Calf Raises - 20 repetitions | **PAGE 24**

Wall Single Leg Circles - 15 repetitions each leg | **PAGE 26**

Wall Table Top - 45 seconds | **PAGE 76**

Wall Leg Raise + Kick Back - 15 repetitions | **PAGE 29**

Wall Scissor - 45 seconds | **PAGE 78**

ADVANCED LEVEL: FLEXIBILITY FOCUS

MONDAY:

Wall Mountain Climbers - 1 minute | **PAGE 20**

Wall Leg Swings - 20 repetitions each leg | **PAGE 22**

Arm Circles - 1 minute | **PAGE 25**

Wall Angels - 20 repetitions | **PAGE 27**

Extended Glute Bridge Rotation - 45 seconds | **PAGE 79**

TUESDAY:

Wall lateral Lunges - 20 repetitions each side | **PAGE 21**

Wall Single-Leg Lifts - 20 repetitions each leg | **PAGE 23**

Knee to Nose - 20 repetitions | **PAGE 28**

Wall Side Leg Lift - 1 minute each side | **PAGE 74**

Dynamic Plank with Wall Support - 45 seconds | **PAGE 80**

WEDNESDAY:

Wall Calf Raises - 25 repetitions | **PAGE 24**

Wall Single Leg Circles - 20 repetitions each leg | **PAGE 26**

Wall Table Top - 1 minute | **PAGE 76**

Wall Leg Raise + Kick Back - 20 repetitions | **PAGE 29**

Wall Scissor - 1 minute | **PAGE 78**

THURSDAY:

Wall Mountain Climbers - 1 minute | **PAGE 20**

Wall Leg Swings - 20 repetitions each leg | **PAGE 22**

Arm Circles - 1 minute | **PAGE 25**

Wall Angels - 20 repetitions | **PAGE 27**

Extended Glute Bridge Rotation - 45 seconds | **PAGE 79**

FRIDAY:

Wall lateral Lunges - 20 repetitions each side | **PAGE 21**

Wall Single-Leg Lifts - 20 repetitions each leg | **PAGE 23**

Knee to Nose - 20 repetitions | **PAGE 28**

Wall Side Leg Lift - 1 minute each side | **PAGE 74**

Dynamic Plank with Wall Support - 45 seconds | **PAGE 80**

SATURDAY:

Wall Calf Raises - 25 repetitions | **PAGE 24**

Wall Single Leg Circles - 20 repetitions each leg | **PAGE 26**

Wall Table Top - 1 minute | **PAGE 76**

Wall Leg Raise + Kick Back - 20 repetitions | **PAGE 29**

Wall Scissor - 1 minute | **PAGE 78**

WEIGHT LOSS WEEKLY WORKOUT PLAN

BEGINNER LEVEL

MONDAY:

Abs And Core Crunch Version - 15 reps (30 calories) | **PAGE 40**

Arm Bends - 20 reps (20 calories) | **PAGE 52**

Wall Hip Thrust - 15 reps (25 calories) | **PAGE 60**

Wall Side Leg Lift - 1 min each side (20 calories) | **PAGE 74**

Wall Table Top - 1 min (15 calories) | **PAGE 76**

Estimated Calories Burned: 110

TUESDAY:

Wall Bicycle Crunches - 20 reps (30 calories) | **PAGE 42**

Wall Push-ups - 15 reps (20 calories) | **PAGE 54**

Lunges classic - 15 reps each leg (25 calories) | **PAGE 61**

Toe Touch Crunch - 1 min (20 calories) | **PAGE 75**

Wall Leg Raise + Kick Back - 15 reps (25 calories) | **PAGE 29**

Estimated Calories Burned: 120

WEDNESDAY:

Abs And Core Oblique Version - 20 reps (35 calories) | **PAGE 41**

Wall Push-ups Dog Pose Version - 20 reps (25 calories) | **PAGE 55**

Lunges + kick back - 20 reps each leg (30 calories) | **PAGE 62**

Wall Single Leg Stretch (Left & Right) - 1 min each (25 calories) | **PAGE 77**

Wall Scissor - 1 min (25 calories) | **PAGE 78**

Estimated Calories Burned: 140

THURSDAY:

Wall Pike Crunches - 20 reps (35 calories) | **PAGE 43**

Wall Touches Plank - 1 min (25 calories) | **PAGE 57**

Wall Squats - 20 reps (30 calories) | **PAGE 64**

Extended Glute Bridge Rotation - 1 min (25 calories) | **PAGE 79**

Dynamic Plank with Wall Support - 1 min (25 calories) | **PAGE 80**

Estimated Calories Burned: 140

FRIDAY:

Wall Abdominal Press Legs Version - 20 reps (35 calories) | **PAGE 44**

Wall Push-ups Dog Pose Version - 20 reps (25 calories) | **PAGE 55**

Wall Sit Heel Raise - 20 reps (30 calories) | **PAGE 65**

Wall Side Leg Lift - 1 min each side (20 calories) | **PAGE 74**

Wall Table Top - 1 min (15 calories) | **PAGE 76**

Estimated Calories Burned: 125

Saturday:

Superman - 1 min (30 calories) | **PAGE 45**

Wall Teaser abs core - 1 min (25 calories) | **PAGE 46**

Wall Walking Plank - 1 min (30 calories) | **PAGE 47**

Dolphin Pose - 1 min (20 calories) | **PAGE 48**

Dolphin Pose with Feet Elevated on Wall - 1 min (25 calories) | **PAGE 49**

Estimated Calories Burned: 130

INTERMEDIATE LEVEL

MONDAY:

Abs And Core Crunch Version - 20 reps (35 calories) | **PAGE 40**

Arm Bends - 25 reps (25 calories) | **PAGE 52**

Wall Hip Thrust - 20 reps (30 calories) | **PAGE 60**

Wall Side Leg Lift - 1.5 min each side (25 calories) | **PAGE 74**

Wall Table Top - 1.5 min (20 calories) | **PAGE 76**

Estimated Calories Burned: 135

TUESDAY:

Wall Bicycle Crunches - 25 reps (35 calories) | **PAGE 42**

Wall Push-ups - 20 reps (25 calories) | **PAGE 54**

Lunges classic - 20 reps each leg (30 calories) | **PAGE 61**

Toe Touch Crunch - 1.5 min (25 calories) | **PAGE 75**

Wall Leg Raise + Kick Back - 20 reps (30 calories) | **PAGE 29**

Estimated Calories Burned: 145

WEDNESDAY:

Abs And Core Oblique Version - 25 reps (40 calories) | **PAGE 41**

Wall Push-ups Dog Pose Version - 25 reps (30 calories) | **PAGE 55**

Lunges + kick back - 25 reps each leg (35 calories) | **PAGE 62**

Wall Single Leg Stretch (Left & Right) - 1 min 30 sec (30 calories) | **PAGE 77**

Wall Scissor - 1 min 30 sec (30 calories) | **PAGE 78**

Estimated Calories Burned: 165

THURSDAY:

Wall Pike Crunches - 25 reps (40 calories) | **PAGE 43**

Wall Touches Plank - 1 min 30 sec (30 calories) | **PAGE 57**

Wall Squats - 25 reps (35 calories) | **PAGE 64**

Extended Glute Bridge Rotation – 1 min 30 sec (30 calories) | **PAGE 79**

Dynamic Plank with Wall Support – 1 min 30 sec (30 calories) | **PAGE 80**

Estimated Calories Burned: 165

FRIDAY:

Wall Abdominal Press Legs Version - 25 reps (40 calories) | **PAGE 44**

Wall Push-ups Dog Pose Version - 25 reps (30 calories) | **PAGE 55**

Wall Sit Heel Raise - 25 reps (35 calories) | **PAGE 65**

Wall Side Leg Lift - 1.5 min each side (25 calories) | **PAGE 74**

Wall Table Top - 1.5 min (20 calories) | **PAGE 76**

Estimated Calories Burned: 150

SATURDAY:

Superman - 1 min 30 sec (35 calories) | **PAGE 45**

Wall Teaser abs core - 1 min 30 sec (30 calories) | **PAGE 46**

Wall Walking Plank - 1 min 30 sec (35 calories) | **PAGE 47**

Dolphin Pose - 1 min 30 sec (25 calories) | **PAGE 48**

Dolphin Pose with Feet Elevated on Wall - 1 min 30 sec (30 calories) | **PAGE 49**

Estimated Calories Burned: 155

ADVANCED LEVEL

MONDAY:

Abs And Core Crunch Version - 30 reps (45 calories) | **PAGE 40**

Arm Bends - 30 reps (30 calories) | **PAGE 52**

Wall Hip Thrust - 25 reps (35 calories) | **PAGE 60**

Wall Side Leg Lift - 2 min each side (30 calories) | **PAGE 74**

Wall Table Top - 2 min (25 calories) | **PAGE 76**

Estimated Calories Burned: 165

TUESDAY:

Wall Bicycle Crunches - 30 reps (45 calories) | **PAGE 42**

Wall Push-ups - 25 reps (30 calories) | **PAGE 54**

Lunges classic - 25 reps each leg (35 calories) | **PAGE 61**

Toe Touch Crunch - 2 min (30 calories) | **PAGE 75**

Wall Leg Raise + Kick Back - 25 reps (35 calories) | **PAGE 29**

Estimated Calories Burned: 175

WEDNESDAY:

Abs And Core Oblique Version - 30 reps (50 calories) | **PAGE 41**

Wall Push-ups Dog Pose Version - 30 reps (35 calories) | **PAGE 55**

Lunges + kick back - 30 reps each leg (40 calories) | **PAGE 62**

Wall Single Leg Stretch (Left & Right) - 2 min each (35 calories) | **PAGE 77**

Wall Scissor - 2 min (35 calories) | **PAGE 78**

Estimated Calories Burned: 195

THURSDAY:

Wall Pike Crunches - 30 reps (50 calories) | **PAGE 43**

Wall Touches Plank - 2 min (35 calories) | **PAGE 57**

Wall Squats - 30 reps (40 calories) | **PAGE 64**

Extended Glute Bridge Rotation - 2 min (35 calories) | **PAGE 79**

Dynamic Plank with Wall Support - 2 min (35 calories) | **PAGE 80**

Estimated Calories Burned: 195

FRIDAY:

Wall Abdominal Press Legs Version - 30 reps (50 calories) | **PAGE 44**

Wall Push-ups Dog Pose Version - 30 reps (35 calories) | **PAGE 55**

Wall Sit Heel Raise - 30 reps (40 calories) | **PAGE 65**

Wall Side Leg Lift - 2 min each side (30 calories) | **PAGE 74**

Wall Table Top - 2 min (25 calories) | **PAGE 76**

Estimated Calories Burned: 180

SATURDAY:

Superman - 2 min (40 calories) | **PAGE 45**

Wall Teaser abs core - 2 min (35 calories) | **PAGE 46**

Wall Walking Plank - 2 min (40 calories) | **PAGE 47**

Dolphin Pose - 2 min (30 calories) | **PAGE 48**

Dolphin Pose with Feet Elevated on Wall - 2 min (35 calories) | **PAGE 49**

Estimated Calories Burned: 180

CORE STRENGHT & FLAT STOMACH FOCUS WEEKLY WORKOUT PLAN

BEGINNER LEVEL

MONDAY:

Abs And Core Crunch Version - 10 reps | **PAGE 40**

Abs And Core Oblique Version - 10 reps | **PAGE 41**

Wall Bicycle Crunches - 10 reps | **PAGE 42**

Wall Hip Thrust - 10 reps | **PAGE 60**

Wall Side Leg Lift - 30 sec each side | **PAGE 74**

TUESDAY:

Wall Pike Crunches - 10 reps | **PAGE 43**

Wall Abdominal Press Legs Version - 10 reps | **PAGE 44**

Superman - 30 sec | **PAGE 45**

Lunges classic - 10 reps each leg | **PAGE 61**

Wall Table Top - 30 sec | **PAGE 76**

WEDNESDAY:

Wall Teaser abs core - 30 sec | **PAGE 46**

Wall Walking Plank - 30 sec | **PAGE 47**

Dolphin Pose - 30 sec | **PAGE 48**

Wall Squats - 10 reps | **PAGE 64**

Wall Sit Heel Raise - 10 reps | **PAGE 65**

THURSDAY:

Reverse Curl - 10 reps | **PAGE 50**

Bridges with Both Legs - 10 reps | **PAGE 60**

Single Leg Bridges - 10 reps | **PAGE 71**

Wall Clamshells - 10 reps | **PAGE 67**

Wall Scissor - 30 sec | **PAGE 78**

FRIDAY:

Wall Abdominal Press Legs Version - 10 reps | **PAGE 44**

Wall Bicycle Crunches - 10 reps | **PAGE 42**

Wall Pike Crunches - 10 reps | **PAGE 43**

Forward Wall Squats - 10 reps | **PAGE 68**

One-Legged Wall Sit - 30 sec | **PAGE 69**

SATURDAY:

Abs And Core Crunch Version - 10 reps | **PAGE 40**

Abs And Core Oblique Version - 10 reps | **PAGE 41**

Wall Teaser abs core - 30 sec | **PAGE 46**

Wall Hip Thrust - 10 reps | **PAGE 60**

Wall Side Leg Lift - 30 sec each side | **PAGE 74**

INTERMEDIATE LEVEL

MONDAY:

Abs And Core Crunch Version - 20 reps | **PAGE 40**

Abs And Core Oblique Version - 20 reps | **PAGE 41**

Wall Bicycle Crunches - 20 reps | **PAGE 42**

Wall Hip Thrust - 20 reps | **PAGE 60**

Wall Side Leg Lift - 1 min each side | **PAGE 74**

TUESDAY:

Wall Pike Crunches - 20 reps | **PAGE 43**

Wall Abdominal Press Legs Version - 20 reps | **PAGE 44**

Superman - 1 min | **PAGE 45**

Lunges classic - 20 reps each leg | **PAGE 61**

Wall Table Top - 1 min | **PAGE 76**

WEDNESDAY:

Wall Teaser abs core - 1 min | **PAGE 46**

Wall Walking Plank - 1 min | **PAGE 47**

Dolphin Pose - 1 min | **PAGE 48**

Wall Squats - 20 reps | **PAGE 64**

Wall Sit Heel Raise - 20 reps | **PAGE 65**

THURSDAY:

Reverse Curl - 20 reps | **PAGE 50**

Bridges with Both Legs - 20 reps | **PAGE 60**

Single Leg Bridges - 20 reps | **PAGE 71**

Wall Clamshells - 20 reps | **PAGE 67**

Wall Scissor - 1 min | **PAGE 78**

FRIDAY:

Wall Abdominal Press Legs Version - 20 reps | **PAGE 44**

Wall Bicycle Crunches - 20 reps | **PAGE 42**

Wall Pike Crunches - 20 reps | **PAGE 43**

Forward Wall Squats - 20 reps | **PAGE 68**

One-Legged Wall Sit - 1 min | **PAGE 69**

SATURDAY:

Abs And Core Crunch Version - 20 reps | **PAGE 40**

Abs And Core Oblique Version - 20 reps | **PAGE 41**

Wall Teaser abs core - 1 min | **PAGE 46**

Wall Hip Thrust - 20 reps | **PAGE 60**

Wall Side Leg Lift - 1 min each side | **PAGE 74**

ADVANCED LEVEL

MONDAY:

Abs And Core Crunch Version - 30 reps | **PAGE 40**

Abs And Core Oblique Version - 30 reps | **PAGE 41**

Wall Bicycle Crunches - 30 reps | **PAGE 42**

Wall Hip Thrust - 25 reps | **PAGE 60**

Wall Side Leg Lift - 2 min each side | **PAGE 74**

TUESDAY:

Wall Pike Crunches - 30 reps | **PAGE 43**

Wall Abdominal Press Legs Version - 30 reps | **PAGE 44**

Superman - 2 min | **PAGE 45**

Lunges classic - 30 reps each leg | **PAGE 61**

Wall Table Top - 2 min | **PAGE 76**

WEDNESDAY:

Wall Teaser abs core - 2 min | **PAGE 46**

Wall Walking Plank - 2 min | **PAGE 47**

Dolphin Pose - 2 min | **PAGE 48**

Wall Squats - 30 reps | **PAGE 64**

Wall Sit Heel Raise - 30 reps | **PAGE 65**

THURSDAY:

Dolphin Pose with Feet Elevated on Wall - 2 min | **PAGE 49**

Reverse Curl - 30 reps | **PAGE 50**

Bridges with Both Legs - 30 reps | **PAGE 60**

Wall Clamshells - 30 reps | **PAGE 67**

Forward Wall Squats - 30 reps | **PAGE 68**

FRIDAY:

Single Leg Bridges - 30 reps each leg | **PAGE 71**

Arm Bends - 30 reps | **PAGE 52**

Wall Push-ups - 30 reps | **PAGE 54**

One-Legged Wall Sit - 2 min | **PAGE 69**

Wall Scissor - 2 min | **PAGE 78**

SATURDAY:

Wall Touches Plank - 2 min | **PAGE 57**

Extended Downward Plank - 2 min | **PAGE 58**

Wall Push-ups Dog Pose Version - 30 reps | **PAGE 55**

Extended Glute Bridge Rotation - 2 min | **PAGE 79**

Dynamic Plank with Wall Support - 2 min | **PAGE 80**

30 DAYS CHALLENGE

BEGINNER LEVEL (DAYS 1-10)

DAY 1:

Abs And Core Crunch Version - 10 reps | **PAGE 40**

Arm Bends - 10 reps | **PAGE 52**

Wall Hip Thrust - 10 reps | **PAGE 60**

Wall Side Leg Lift - 30 sec each side | **PAGE 74**

Wall Table Top - 30 sec | **PAGE 76**

DAY 2:

Abs And Core Oblique Version - 10 reps | **PAGE 41**

Arms/Shoulder Stretch - 30 sec | **PAGE 53**

Lunges classic - 10 reps each leg | **PAGE 61**

Toe Touch Crunch - 10 reps | **PAGE 75**

Wall Leg Raise + Kick Back - 10 reps | **PAGE 29**

DAY 3:

Wall Bicycle Crunches - 10 reps | **PAGE 42**

Wall Push-ups - 10 reps | **PAGE 54**

Lunges + kick back - 10 reps each leg | **PAGE 62**

Wall Single Leg Stretch (Left & Right) - 10 reps each | **PAGE 77**

Wall Scissor - 30 sec | **PAGE 78**

DAY 4:

Wall Pike Crunches - 10 reps | **PAGE 43**

Wall Push-ups Dog Pose Version - 10 reps | **PAGE 55**

Back to the wall Lunges - 10 reps each leg | **PAGE 63**

Extended Glute Bridge Rotation - 10 reps | **PAGE 79**

Dynamic Plank with Wall Support - 30 sec | **PAGE 80**

DAY 5:

Wall Abdominal Press Legs Version - 10 reps | **PAGE 44**

Seated Trunk Rotation - 10 reps each side | **PAGE 56**

Wall Squats - 10 reps | **PAGE 64**

Wall Side Leg Lift - 30 sec each side | **PAGE 74**

Wall Table Top - 30 sec | **PAGE 76**

DAY 6:

Superman - 30 sec | **PAGE 45**

Wall Touches Plank - 30 sec | **PAGE 57**

Wall Sit Heel Raise - 10 reps | **PAGE 65**

Toe Touch Crunch - 10 reps | **PAGE 75**

Wall Leg Raise + Kick Back - 10 reps | **PAGE 29**

DAY 7:

Wall Teaser abs core - 30 sec | **PAGE 46**

Extended Downward Plank - 30 sec | **PAGE 58**

Standing Wall Leg Lifts - 10 reps each leg | **PAGE 66**

Wall Single Leg Stretch (Left & Right) - 10 reps each | **PAGE 77**

Wall Scissor - 30 sec | **PAGE 78**

DAY 8:

Wall Walking Plank - 30 sec | **PAGE 47**

Arm Bends - 10 reps | **PAGE 52**

Wall Clamshells - 10 reps each leg | **PAGE 67**

Extended Glute Bridge Rotation - 10 reps | **PAGE 79**

Dynamic Plank with Wall Support - 30 sec | **PAGE 80**

DAY 9:

Dolphin Pose - 30 sec | **PAGE 48**

Arms/Shoulder Stretch - 30 sec | **PAGE 53**

Forward Wall Squats - 10 reps | **PAGE 68**

Wall Side Leg Lift - 30 sec each side | **PAGE 74**

Wall Table Top - 30 sec | **PAGE 76**

DAY 10:

Dolphin Pose with Feet Elevated on Wall - 30 sec | **PAGE 49**

Wall Push-ups - 10 reps | **PAGE 54**

One-Legged Wall Sit - 30 sec | **PAGE 69**

Toe Touch Crunch - 10 reps | **PAGE 75**

Wall Leg Raise + Kick Back - 10 reps | **PAGE 29**

INTERMEDIATE LEVEL (DAYS 11-20)

DAY 11:

Abs And Core Crunch Version - 20 reps | **PAGE 40**

Arm Bends - 20 reps | **PAGE 52**

Wall Hip Thrust - 20 reps | **PAGE 60**

Wall Side Leg Lift - 1 min each side | **PAGE 74**

Wall Table Top - 1 min | **PAGE 76**

DAY 12:

Abs And Core Oblique Version - 20 reps | **PAGE 41**

Arms/Shoulder Stretch - 1 min | **PAGE 53**

Lunges classic - 20 reps each leg | **PAGE 61**

Toe Touch Crunch - 20 reps | **PAGE 75**

Wall Leg Raise + Kick Back - 20 reps | **PAGE 29**

DAY 13:

Wall Bicycle Crunches - 20 reps | **PAGE 42**

Wall Push-ups - 20 reps | **PAGE 54**

Lunges + kick back - 20 reps each leg | **PAGE 62**

Wall Single Leg Stretch (Left & Right) - 20 reps each | **PAGE 77**

Wall Scissor - 1 min | **PAGE 78**

DAY 14:

Wall Pike Crunches - 20 reps | **PAGE 43**

Wall Push-ups Dog Pose Version - 20 reps | **PAGE 55**

Back to the wall Lunges - 20 reps each leg | **PAGE 63**

Extended Glute Bridge Rotation - 20 reps | **PAGE 79**

Dynamic Plank with Wall Support - 1 min | **PAGE 80**

DAY 15:

Wall Abdominal Press Legs Version - 20 reps | **PAGE 44**

Seated Trunk Rotation - 20 reps each side | **PAGE 56**

Wall Squats - 20 reps | **PAGE 64**

Wall Side Leg Lift - 1 min each side | **PAGE 74**

Wall Table Top - 1 min | **PAGE 76**

DAY 16:

Superman - 1 min | **PAGE 45**

Wall Touches Plank - 1 min | **PAGE 57**

Wall Sit Heel Raise - 20 reps | **PAGE 65**

Toe Touch Crunch - 20 reps | **PAGE 75**

Wall Leg Raise + Kick Back - 20 reps | **PAGE 29**

DAY 17:

Wall Teaser abs core - 1 min | **PAGE 46**

Extended Downward Plank - 1 min | **PAGE 58**

Standing Wall Leg Lifts - 20 reps each leg | **PAGE 66**

Wall Single Leg Stretch (Left & Right) - 20 reps each | **PAGE 77**

Wall Scissor - 1 min | **PAGE 78**

DAY 18:

Wall Walking Plank - 1 min | **PAGE 47**

Arm Bends - 20 reps | **PAGE 52**

Wall Clamshells - 20 reps each leg | **PAGE 67**

Extended Glute Bridge Rotation - 20 reps | **PAGE 79**

Dynamic Plank with Wall Support - 1 min | **PAGE 80**

DAY 19:

Dolphin Pose - 1 min | **PAGE 48**

Arms/Shoulder Stretch - 1 min | **PAGE 53**

Forward Wall Squats - 20 reps | **PAGE 68**

Wall Side Leg Lift - 1 min each side | **PAGE 74**

Wall Table Top - 1 min | **PAGE 76**

DAY 20:

Dolphin Pose with Feet Elevated on Wall - 1 min | **PAGE 49**

Wall Push-ups - 20 reps | **PAGE 54**

One-Legged Wall Sit - 1 min | **PAGE 69**

Toe Touch Crunch - 20 reps | **PAGE 75**

Wall Leg Raise + Kick Back - 20 reps | **PAGE 29**

ADVANCED LEVEL (DAYS 21-30)

DAY 21:

Abs And Core Crunch Version - 30 reps | **PAGE 40**

Arm Bends - 30 reps | **PAGE 52**

Wall Hip Thrust - 30 reps | **PAGE 60**

Wall Side Leg Lift - 1 min 30 sec each side | **PAGE 74**

Wall Table Top - 1 min 30 sec | **PAGE 76**

DAY 22:

Abs And Core Oblique Version - 30 reps | **PAGE 41**

Arms/Shoulder Stretch - 1 min 30 sec | **PAGE 53**

Lunges classic - 30 reps each leg | **PAGE 61**

Toe Touch Crunch - 30 reps | **PAGE 75**

Wall Leg Raise + Kick Back - 30 reps | **PAGE 29**

DAY 23:

Wall Bicycle Crunches - 30 reps | **PAGE 42**

Wall Push-ups - 30 reps | **PAGE 54**

Lunges + kick back - 30 reps each leg | **PAGE 62**

Wall Single Leg Stretch (Left & Right) - 30 reps each | **PAGE 77**

Wall Scissor - 1 min 30 sec | **PAGE 78**

DAY 24:

Wall Pike Crunches - 30 reps | **PAGE 43**

Wall Push-ups Dog Pose Version - 30 reps | **PAGE 55**

Back to the wall Lunges - 30 reps each leg | **PAGE 63**

Extended Glute Bridge Rotation - 30 reps | **PAGE 79**

Dynamic Plank with Wall Support - 1 min 30 sec | **PAGE 80**

DAY 25:

Wall Abdominal Press Legs Version - 30 reps | **PAGE 44**

Seated Trunk Rotation - 30 reps each side | **PAGE 56**

Wall Squats - 30 reps | **PAGE 64**

Wall Side Leg Lift - 1 min 30 sec each side | **PAGE 74**

Wall Table Top - 1 min 30 sec | **PAGE 76**

DAY 26:

Superman - 1 min 30 sec | **PAGE 45**

Wall Touches Plank - 1 min 30 sec | **PAGE 57**

Wall Sit Heel Raise - 30 reps | **PAGE 65**

Toe Touch Crunch - 30 reps | **PAGE 75**

Wall Leg Raise + Kick Back - 30 reps | **PAGE 29**

DAY 27:

Wall Teaser abs core - 1 min 30 sec | **PAGE 46**

Extended Downward Plank - 1 min 30 sec | **PAGE 58**

Standing Wall Leg Lifts - 30 reps each leg | **PAGE 66**

Wall Single Leg Stretch (Left & Right) - 30 reps each | **PAGE 77**

Wall Scissor - 1 min 30 sec | **PAGE 78**

DAY 28:

Wall Walking Plank - 1 min 30 sec | **PAGE 47**

Arm Bends - 30 reps | **PAGE 52**

Wall Clamshells - 30 reps each leg | **PAGE 67**

Extended Glute Bridge Rotation - 30 reps | **PAGE 79**

Dynamic Plank with Wall Support - 1 min 30 sec | **PAGE 80**

DAY 29:

Dolphin Pose - 1 min 30 sec | **PAGE 48**

Arms/Shoulder Stretch - 1 min 30 sec | **PAGE 53**

Forward Wall Squats - 30 reps | **PAGE 68**

Wall Side Leg Lift - 1 min 30 sec each side | **PAGE 74**

Wall Table Top - 1 min 30 sec | **PAGE 76**

DAY 30:

Dolphin Pose with Feet Elevated on Wall - 1 min 30 sec | **PAGE 49**

Wall Push-ups - 30 reps | **PAGE 54**

One-Legged Wall Sit - 1 min 30 sec | **PAGE 69**

Toe Touch Crunch - 30 reps | **PAGE 75**

Wall Leg Raise + Kick Back - 30 reps | **PAGE 29**

Chapter 6: Nutrition and Well-being

Nutrition Tips for Optimal Performance in Wall Pilates

In the realm of Wall Pilates, where precision, strength, and flexibility converge, nutrition plays a pivotal role in determining one's performance. To fuel the body adequately for this unique exercise regimen, it's essential to prioritize a balanced intake of macronutrients. Carbohydrates, often dubbed the body's primary energy source, should be consumed in the form of whole grains and complex sources to provide sustained energy for prolonged sessions against the wall. Proteins, vital for muscle repair and growth, should be derived from lean sources like poultry, fish, legumes, and tofu. Healthy fats from avocados, nuts, and olive oil can aid in joint lubrication and inflammation reduction. Hydration, too, cannot be overlooked; maintaining optimal fluid levels ensures muscle function and aids in post-exercise recovery. Moreover, micronutrients like magnesium and calcium, found in leafy greens and dairy, respectively, can bolster bone strength, a crucial aspect of Wall Pilates. By integrating these nutritional guidelines, practitioners can enhance their stamina, reduce injury risk, and truly harness the transformative power of Wall Pilates.

Macronutrients:

1. Carbohydrates:

Whole Grains (e.g., quinoa, brown rice, oats): Provide sustained energy and are rich in fiber, aiding digestion.
Sweet Potatoes: A great source of complex carbs and vitamin A.
Fruits (e.g., bananas, berries, apples): Offer quick energy and are packed with vitamins and antioxidants.

Legumes (e.g., lentils, chickpeas, beans): High in fiber and protein, supporting prolonged energy and muscle function.

2. Proteins:

Chicken Breast: A lean source of protein that supports muscle growth and repair.
Fish (e.g., salmon, mackerel, sardines): Rich in omega-3 fatty acids and protein, promoting heart health and muscle recovery.
Tofu: A plant-based protein source that also provides essential amino acids.
Eggs: Offer high-quality protein and essential vitamins and minerals.

3. Fats:

Avocados: Provide healthy monounsaturated fats and are rich in potassium.
Nuts (e.g., almonds, walnuts, cashews): Offer healthy fats, protein, and essential minerals.
Olive Oil: Contains heart-healthy monounsaturated fats and antioxidants.
Chia Seeds: A source of omega-3 fatty acids, fiber, and protein.

Micronutrients and Their Sources:

1. Calcium: Essential for bone health.

Sources: Dairy products (milk, cheese, yogurt), fortified plant-based milk, leafy greens, and sardines.

2. Iron: Vital for oxygen transport in the blood.

Sources: Red meat, spinach, lentils, pumpkin seeds, and fortified cereals.

3. Magnesium: Supports muscle function and energy production.

Sources: Almonds, spinach, avocado, and dark chocolate.

4. Potassium: Regulates fluid balance and muscle contractions.

Sources: Bananas, sweet potatoes, beans, and spinach.

5. Vitamin C: Important for immune function and skin health.

Sources: Oranges, strawberries, bell peppers, and broccoli.

6. Vitamin D: Essential for calcium absorption and bone health.

Sources: Fatty fish, fortified dairy products, egg yolks, and sunlight exposure.

7. Zinc: Supports immune function and wound healing.

Sources: Beef, chickpeas, cashews, and pumpkin seeds.

8. Folate: Vital for DNA synthesis and cell division.

Sources: Leafy greens, fortified cereals, oranges, and legumes.

Weight Management: Weight Loss, Maintenance, And Muscle Growth.

To achieve one of these goals, it is essential to know your basal metabolism, which, in simple terms, is the amount of calories your body burns every day.

Your basal metabolism rate is produced through the following basal metabolic rate formula:
Women: BMR = 447.593 + (9.247 x weight in kg) + (3.098 x height in cm) – (4.330 x age in years)

If you don't like math, I created an Excel table just for it.

SCAN THE QR CODE

INSTRUCTIONS: To fill out the table above, you need to click on 'File' and then click on 'Make a Copy'

In addition to this, to achieve your physical goal, other factors such as how much movement you do during the day must be considered.

For this very reason, I decided to share with you this website where you can calculate for free the amount of calories you need to lose weight, maintain it, or increase it.

SCAN THE QR CODE

Conclusion

As we come to the close of this guide, I want to extend my heartfelt gratitude to you. Your commitment to embarking on this Wall Pilates journey, and your trust in this guide, is truly commendable. Remember, every page you turned, every exercise you tried, and every moment you dedicated to your well-being is a testament to your determination and passion.

It's not just about the physical transformation; it's about the mental and emotional growth you've nurtured throughout this process. You should be incredibly proud of yourself. Not everyone takes the initiative to better themselves, but you did. And that speaks volumes about your character and dedication.

As you continue on this path, always remember that the journey is just as important, if not more so, than the destination. Celebrate your small victories, learn from the challenges, and always strive to be the best version of yourself.

Thank you for allowing me to be a part of your transformative journey. Stay motivated, stay strong, and always remember to be proud of every step you take towards a healthier, happier you.

With warmest regards and best wishes for your continued success,

Eva Ross

YOUR OPINION IS INVALUABLE!

If you have a moment, I would be very grateful if you could leave a review, sharing your outcomes and thoughts on this book. Your insights will help other readers and also provide significant input for me in writing future books.

SCAN THE QR CODE BELOW TO LEAVE A REVIEW

Printed in Great Britain
by Amazon